SECOND EDITION

RESTRAINT AND SECLUSION

Improving Practice and Maintaining JCAHO Compliance

Jack Zusman, MD

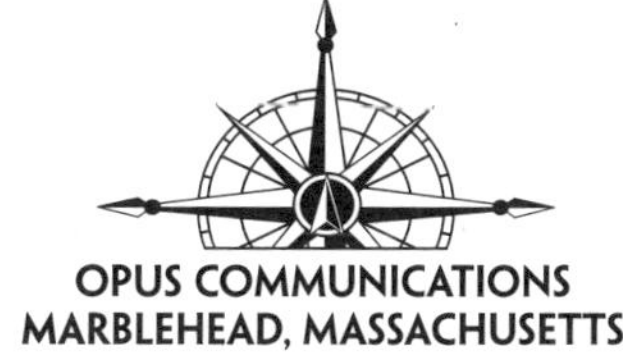

OPUS COMMUNICATIONS
MARBLEHEAD, MASSACHUSETTS

Restraint and Seclusion: Improving Practice and Maintaining JCAHO Compliance is published by Opus Communications, Inc.

 5 4 3 2 1

ISBN 1–57839–071–0

Opus Communications provides information resources for the healthcare industry. A selected listing of other newsletters and books is found in the back of this book.

Opus Communications is not affiliated in any way with the Joint Commission on Accreditation of Healthcare Organizations.

Jennifer Cofer, Executive Publisher
Rob Stuart, Publisher
Jack Zusman, MD, Author
Kristen Woods, Executive Editor
Jim Fiebelkorn, Assistant Editor
John Devins, Contributing Editor
Jean St. Pierre, Creative Director
Tom Philbrook, Cover Designer
Cynthia Cross, Graphic Artist
Mike Mirabello, Graphic Artist

Advice given is general. Readers should consult professional counsel for specific legal, ethical, or clinical questions. Arrangements can be made for quantity discounts.

For more information, contact:

Opus Communications
P.O. Box 1168
Marblehead, MA 01945
Telephone: 800/650-6787 or 781/639-1872
Fax: 781/639-2982
E-mail: customer_service@opuscomm.com

Visit the Opus Communications World Wide Web site: http://www.opuscomm.com

TABLE OF CONTENTS

About the Author

Jack Zusman, MD is a psychiatrist and a recognized expert, author, and lecturer in the healthcare industry. He has practical experience as a clinician in psychiatric hospitals and mental health centers and as a CEO of a freestanding psychiatric facility.

Dr. Zusman serves as a consultant to a number of other healthcare organizations, and is a licensed health care risk manager in the state of Florida. He serves as an associate in risk management with the Insurance Institute of America, and is a professor at the Florida Mental Health Institute, University of South Florida. In addition, Dr. Zusman is certified by the American Board of Psychiatry and Neurology and the American Board of Preventive Medicine.

Preface

Editor's note: This book is the second edition of Restraint and Seclusion: Improving Practice and Maintaining JCAHO Compliance. *The first edition was published in September 1996. For the benefit of readers who do not have a copy of the first edition, we include the Preface material from the first edition below, in its entirety, as well as material that Dr. Zusman wrote specifically for this second edition. Note that references to the JCAHO standards and other timely discussions in the original Preface material are now out of date; Dr. Zusman's new Preface material and the rest of this book provide current information.*

A book about restraints? Why would anyone need that? Just because the Joint Commission on Accreditation of Healthcare Organizations (JCAHO) changed its standards a little bit, who needs a book about something that is no more than common sense?

A lot of people feel that way, and I used to also. That feeling is undoubtedly one of the reasons why over 50% of the hospitals surveyed by the JCAHO in the first half of 1995 received Type I recommendations (compliance scores indicating a need for immediate improvement) relating to the standard on restraint or seclusion (TX.7.1), and the trend is continuing in 1996.

Years ago, when I was a psychiatric resident (in those days, the residents ran the clinical units), restraint use was just a regular part of psychiatric hospital life, like eating in the cafeteria or going on rounds in the morning. We had patients put into restraint (or sometimes seclusion) without a second thought and whenever it seemed appropriate. Very little consideration was involved in decisions regarding restraint, and everyone around the hospital (including the patients, we hoped) knew that if a patient acted "crazy" enough, he or she was likely to be restrained.

As far as my resident colleagues and I knew, ordering restraint was something any doctor could do whenever he or she thought it was appropriate—just like ordering aspirin for a fever—and the nurses would do whatever was necessary to get a patient restrained. We never had any formal instruction about restraint, and we never thought about what it might mean to a patient to be restrained. There probably was some protocol or set of instructions for the nurses to follow when they applied restraints, but we doctors did not know or care about it.

Back then, nurses sometimes decided on their own to restrain patients, and they got doctors' signatures on the patient records to ratify their decisions only after (sometimes many hours after) patients were restrained. Patients sometimes spent days in restraint or seclusion, and it was considered routine for patients or staff to get hurt during the process of applying restraint. When patients occasionally complained to us that particular nurses were using restraints or seclusion inappropriately, such as for punishment, we doctors didn't believe them.

I also worked on medical wards many years ago and remember that residents on medical, surgical, and pediatric wards were even less concerned about restraint use than residents on psychiatric wards. And why should they be concerned? Residents on medical and pediatric wards believed they never used restraint and that restraint was something used only in psychiatric units.

In truth, residents on medical, surgical, and pediatric wards never ordered restraints, but frequently encountered patients who were tied to their beds and chairs because nurses had decided that such ties were necessary. On pediatric wards, many patients were tied in some way to prevent them from pulling out a tube, disturbing a dressing, or climbing out of bed. But the residents felt that tying a patient into bed or restricting a patient's hand movement was done only when the need was obvious, and since it was for the patient's own good, why make a big deal of it?

Even today, I sometimes encounter people who think this way about restraint. But my experiences and reading have changed the way I think about restraint. I share many of the things I have learned about restraint in this book.

This book attempts to help organizations define the terms *restraint* and *seclusion* in a way that meets the JCAHO standards and ensures that all uses of restraint and seclusion are handled appropriately. It also discusses common uses of restraint and seclusion, problems and issues associated with restraint and seclusion, and advice for decreasing and improving restraint use. Because the JCAHO came out with 25 new restraint standards for hospitals, behavioral healthcare settings, and ambulatory care settings (effective July 1, 1996 and continuing unchanged at least through 1997), two chapters of this book are devoted to discussing what these new standards require, how they will be surveyed and scored, and what organizations need to do to ensure compliance with the standards. Finally, since organizational plans, policies, and procedures are critical to proper restraint and seclusion use, this book discusses and offers samples of these documents.

Readers should note that this book does not intend to provide legal advice; organizations should consult appropriate legal counsel when necessary. In many states, restraint use is regulated by state law or regulation, so readers must be aware of state requirements before making changes to their restraint policies.

This book also does not represent the official opinion of the JCAHO; it is an entirely separate guidebook that is best used alongside the appropriate JCAHO accreditation manual. Although this book is most directly relevant to hospitals, behavioral healthcare facilities, and ambulatory care settings (which share some of the new JCAHO restraint standards), many discussions are relevant to other types of facilities as well, such as long-term care and home care facilities. For the sake of simplicity, this book often refers to hospitals, but the information is equally relevant to behavioral health care and ambulatory care. And sometimes the book uses the term organizations to cover all relevant types of facilities.

Generally, restraint and seclusion are not dealt with separately in this book; the term *restraint* is intended to apply to seclusion as well. The JCAHO treats restraint and seclusion together, as do most regulatory bodies, and the two procedures have much in common. When separate consideration is appropriate, this book does discuss restraint and seclusion separately.

This book reports on all that is known regarding the JCAHO's interpretation of its restraint and seclusion standards and approaches to surveying compliance at the time of its publication (September 1996). Clearly, there are still some unanswered questions. Readers regularly should check the JCAHO's newsletter, *Perspectives*, and Opus Communications' newsletter, *Briefings on JCAHO*, for any further developments.

On a personal note, I want to thank Kristen Woods, my editor at Opus Communications, for her dedication and assistance throughout the preparation of this book. I also want to thank the Resource Center staff at the JCAHO and the library staff at Florida Mental Health Institute, University of South Florida, for their assistance in bibliographic searches. Finally, I want to thank many colleagues at the JCAHO and in the hospitals and other facilities I have visited for sharing information with me.

One of the things I have learned in many years as a clinician and administrator in healthcare organizations is that there are no final answers to many of the questions with which we constantly struggle. I welcome comments, corrections, suggestions, or additional information from readers. Please write to me at Opus Communications, P.O. Box 1168, Marblehead, MA 01945.

Preface to the second edition

Major and unexpected changes to the JCAHO standards and HCFA hospital *Conditions of Participation (COP)* standards for restraint and seclusion have compelled us to undertake a new edition of this book. In addition to discussing the latest information regarding the JCAHO and the COP, we have taken advantage of the opportunity to make some additions and revisions that we hope will make the book more useful.

I wrote the first edition right after the July 1, 1996, restraint and seclusion standards were announced but before they had gone into effect. At that time, it was impossible to know how the fine points of some of the standards were going to be interpreted and how the surveyors were going to evaluate compliance. Since then, we have all accumulated a good deal of experience with these issues. Furthermore—no doubt because of the considerably increased emphasis JCAHO has forced hospitals to place on regulating and monitoring restraint and seclusion use—we know a lot more about how hospitals improve their restraint and seclusion practices. We have incorporated this new knowledge into the second edition.

Unfortunately, the need to make educated guesses about standards interpretation and surveyor behavior is still a problem for this second edition. All 25 of the 1996 restraint and seclusion standards have been renumbered, and many of them have been rewritten. And 29 standards have replaced the 25. Although 21 of the standards are very similar to previous standards and, therefore, presumably will be officially interpreted and evaluated exactly as the previous ones, eight of them are new. Most of the new standards are similar both to previous standards and to some of the 21 other new standards, but there are a few that are completely new.

Additionally, the group of eight standards represents a change in the JCAHO's approach. The 1996 standards, for the most part, were exactly the same for acute care general hospitals (and other acute care organizations such as ambulatory surgery centers) as for behavioral healthcare organizations. Now there are standards that apply either to the first category or to the second, but not to both. Only as experience accumulates will we know exactly the impact of this changed approach.

In any case, interpretation of standards and surveyor practices change all the time, although admittedly often to an imperceptible degree. Surveyors even change their application of standards that remain unchanged for years in their written form. Nothing is final or definitive in the JCAHO world (just the same as in the big world). We can only do our best to make predictions that are based on the past, and the future will always surprise us.

As in the first edition, we have attempted to go well beyond JCAHO requirements to consider and make recommendations regarding good clinical practice. There are many positive results from the JCAHO's effort to make standards less prescriptive and more flexible so as to meet the needs of each hospital or other organization. One of the negative results, though, is that it is no longer safe for organizations to be satisfied and feel that there can be no grounds for an accusation that they did not meet accepted standards of care once they comply with all of the JCAHO standards. In a number of areas—and restraint and seclusion is certainly one of them—the standard of care seems to be more stringent than JCAHO standards require. (Incidentally, another important reason to go beyond the minimum necessary to achieve compliance with the JCAHO standards is surveyor variability. What might seem like reasonable and acceptable compliance to one surveyor [or consultant or outside observer] might appear unsatisfactory to another surveyor. Logic suggests that it is safer to be well beyond the minimum.)

In the first edition, we emphasized the danger of using restraint. In brief, we suggest that restraint be considered analogous to open-heart surgery: probably lifesaving when absolutely necessary, but not something to be undertaken lightly or before less dangerous alternatives have been tried and failed. Since the first edition, the JCAHO has begun systematically collecting and analyzing data on "sentinel events"—serious adverse occurrences that accredited organizations are required to report to the JCAHO. A significant portion of those events relates to restraint use, and recently JCAHO published *Sentinel Event Alert #8*, which reported the dangers of restraint.

As was the first edition, this book is the result of the work of a number of persons and their organizations. I want to acknowledge their contributions and thank them. Opus Communications—in particular, Kristen Woods, who has now become Executive Editor, and John Devins and Jim Fiebelkorn, editors, have of course been major contributors of support. At the JCAHO, the Resource Center staffed by Jan Aleccia and Laura Shedore, my fellow surveyor, Elizabeth D. Geffers, Ann Kobs, who was one of the stalwarts of standards interpretation and is now an expert on sentinel events, and Pat Staten in standards interpretation, have been very helpful. At the University of South Florida, the administration of the Florida Mental Health Institute has made time available to me to do this book, as well as a host of related activities. Finally, I want to offer the most thanks to various hospitals and their staff members (who obviously can't be named) for the many opportunities to observe restraint and seclusion in action, to discuss problems and alternatives, and to share sources of additional information.

New in 1999:

Federal Standards on Restraint and Seclusion in Hospitals

Introduction

As the second edition of *Restraint and Seclusion* was nearing completion, I was surprised to learn that the federal government was about to establish standards for restraint and seclusion use in hospitals. This would occur through the Health Care Financing Administration's (HCFA) issuing amended *Conditions of Participation* (COP) for Hospitals. Such an event was indeed big news.

Up until now, the federal government had been content to leave monitoring of many details of hospital operation—including the application of restraint or seclusion—to the Joint Commission on Accreditation of Healthcare Organizations (JCAHO) and the state governments. And although many of the state governments had laws or regulations dealing with restraint and seclusion, they typically followed the JCAHO standards. Thus the JCAHO standards on restraint and seclusion set the pattern for the hospital industry. (This is different from the situation in the long-term care or nursing home industry, in which HCFA has had restraint requirements for a number of years, JCAHO is not so dominant, and the importance of payments from Medicare and Medicaid in long-term care make HCFA an important regulator.)

Now there are federally established restraint and seclusion standards for hospitals. And, most importantly, these standards appear to differ in several key aspects from the latest JCAHO standards.

All of this happened at a time when there was great national concern with possible improper use of restraint in hospitals and a campaign to increase monitoring and performance quality. The new federal standards were instituted on extremely short notice (announced in late June 1999 and effective August 2), suggesting some pressure to get them out. The document announcing the standards provided no information about exactly how stringently the standards are to be enforced, or about who will enforce them. (Currently, HCFA carries out relatively few hospital inspections itself; JCAHO surveyors do most of the hospital visits. But JCAHO surveyors are not trained to evaluate those HCFA requirements that differ from JCAHO standards, as portions of the new standards most certainly do. (See Figure B, p. 17 for a summary of COP requirements that differ from the JCAHO requirements.)

Faced with the problem of a book about to go to press and a development that is extremely relevant to the book, but that leaves many questions about the development still unanswered, Opus Communications and I had a dilemma. Do we ignore the HCFA standards, or do we incorporate them into this second edition, doing our best to estimate how some of the elements will play out? We chose the latter course, but decided not to rewrite any of the book and instead to add the following section that can stand alone. The following section provides the best information we have as the new HCFA COP standards take effect on August 2, 1999.

Sometimes circumstances force a decision in the absence of sufficient information. This is one of those situations. Our best estimate is that the new standards will take effect on August 2, 1999 and that the final standards that will eventually replace these "interim final" standards will be very similar. We also estimate that JCAHO will either modify its own standards to resemble the federal ones or that JCAHO will train and require the surveyors to evaluate compliance with the federal ones.

Furthermore, however this gets settled, it will not happen very soon. After HCFA obtains all its public comments (the public has until September 2, 1999 to comment), it will take some time to digest them. Then it will have to write and promulgate clarifying definitions, interpretive guidelines, and final standards. Meanwhile, JCAHO will probably wait to see what is going to happen and then take whatever action it deems to be appropriate. JCAHO typically takes one to two years between the time it issues a draft of a possible new standard and the point at which the standard becomes effective. So we may be two or three years away from federal and JCAHO restraint and seclusion standards that coincide and are consistently enforced. All of this estimation helped us to arrive at the decision to publish now rather than wait.

Readers should carefully watch for announcements of developments regarding this situation. Many of the Opus Communications newsletters will carry stories about it, and readers may obtain information through the direct link to this title on the Opus Communications web site, <www.opuscomm.com>.

As with all the rest of this book, Kristen Woods at Opus has been a great help in preparing and editing the material.

—Jack Zusman

New COP more stringent than JCAHO 1999 standards

On July 2, 1999, the Health Care Financing Administration (HCFA) published an interim final rule regarding patients' rights in the Medicare/Medicaid *Conditions of Participation (COP)* for hospitals.[1] The patients' rights requirements include significant new standards dealing with restraint and seclusion. All hospitals serving Medicare- or Medicaid-funded patients will have to comply with these standards effective August 2, 1999.

According to the explanation accompanying the document, 4,734 of the 6,163 hospitals involved are JCAHO-accredited. Although the new standards considerably overlap the JCAHO standards, they do not coincide 100%. Because the new standards are interim final, there is still a possibility of change; however, the standards have been under study for some time and the likelihood of change seems small. Furthermore, were changes to occur, quite likely it would be many months before they would be announced and be in effect. In the meantime, the interim final standards prevail.

At present (July, 1999) there is as yet no experience with the enforcement of these changes, so the material below is based only on best guesses. We have decided to go to press at this point rather than wait until more information is available because readers need timely information on the primary focus of this book—the new 1999 JCAHO standards. It likely will be six months or more before we know the impact of the new COP, and that will be too long to delay this book. Information about the COP enforcement will be published in Opus Communications newsletters as soon as it is available, and the next edition of this book will contain a comprehensive review of the COP.

Interaction of COP and the JCAHO

JCAHO surveyors' attitudes toward the COP requirements that are different from or go beyond the JCAHO standards remain to be seen. Two JCAHO standards (GO.2.4 and MA.2) deal with compliance with applicable law and regulation. A Medicare-approved hospital's failure to comply with some part of the COP that is not required by the JCAHO standards could lead to noncompliance scores on

[1] This document is in *The Federal Register*, July 2, 1999, Volume 64, Number 127, pages 36069–36089.

either or both of these standards. But at present, JCAHO surveyors do not systematically go beyond JCAHO standards to evaluate compliance with the existing COP or any other state or federal requirements.

Although only those those hospitals wishing to be reimbursed for treating Medicare/Medicaid patients must comply with the COP, the impact of the new COP requirements is likely to be broader. First, hospitals that must comply with the COP must do so not only for Medicare/Medicaid patients, but for *all* patients. Second, state licensing authorities and the JCAHO will likely consider strengthening their own requirements to coincide with those of the new COP.

The brief analysis of the COP standards relating to restraint and seclusion that we offer here is based only on reading the COP. Many issues and definitions of terms remain to be clarified. In the discussion below, we do not attempt to deal with every one of these issues remaining to be clarified, but only the more significant ones.

What is the COP?

The *Conditions of Participation* is a set of standards that all Medicare/Medicaid participating organizations must meet. There is a COP for each type of organization. The COP we discuss here is the one for hospitals—specifically, "short-term, psychiatric, rehabilitation, long-term, children's, and alcohol-drug." Technically, an organization's license determines whether it is a hospital.

Representatives of agencies with which HCFA contracts, rather than HCFA employees directly, usually evaluate organizations' compliance with the COP. Typically, the contracted agency in any state is the state licensing authority. Hospitals that are accredited by the JCAHO or the American Osteopathic Association (AOA) are exempt from routine HCFA inspections, since JCAHO or AOA accreditation is "deemed" to meet HCFA requirements. But hospitals that have no interest in JCAHO or AOA accreditation undergo HCFA surveys and need to meet the COP standards to meet the requirements for participation in Medicare and Medicaid. HCFA also carries out "validation surveys"—surveys that check on the JCAHO and AOA survey processes—at a small sample of accredited facilities. A hospital that is subject to a validation survey can receive noncompliance penalties, regardless of the findings of its JCAHO or AOA survey. Consensus among those familiar with both the COP and JCAHO requirements seems to be that there is at best an 80% overlap between the requirements of the two organizations.

The new COP restraint and seclusion standards

There are five new patients' rights standards, of which two relate to restraint (see Figure A, p. 14 for the text of the new hospital COP restraint standards). Until now, there have not been *any* standards in the hospital COP relating to restraint or seclusion, although there have been such standards in the COP for long-term care. In the absence of hospital COP standards, the JCAHO and the individual states have had the major responsibility of establishing and enforcing minimum requirements for restraint and seclusion use. (Generally, the states have modeled their requirements on the JCAHO's, but a number of states have not yet incorporated the changes in the 1996 JCAHO standards; so it will be even longer before the 1999 JCAHO standards have an effect on all the states.)

General points about the COP standards

As with any set of standards, a certain amount of discretion is left to the individual evaluating compliance. JCAHO assists its surveyors by expanding and explaining the standards through accompanying intent statements and scoring guidelines. HCFA offers a document, *Hospitals Interpretive Guidelines and Survey Procedures*, for the same purpose. The portion of the guidelines covering the new restraint standards is not yet available. And even when it is available, the details of which steps a hospital should take to ensure compliance with the COP will not be certain; hospitals will not know for sure until experience with surveying the new COP standards accumulates.

A complicating factor in knowing exactly what the new COP standards mean in practice is that most of the hospitals subject to the COP standards will not be reviewed by HCFA surveyors applying the standards. Because of deemed status, JCAHO surveyors will survey the hospitals applying the JCAHO restraint and seclusion standards. There are some important differences between current JCAHO standards and the new COP standards (we discuss these differences below).

A final point to keep in mind is that, as we said above, because the present version of the COP standards is "interim final," it is still possible (although not likely) that the final version will contain further changes.

Comparing the new COP and JCAHO 1999 medical and surgical restraint standards

Much of both sets of standards is essentially the same, although the style of presentation and precise wording differ. However, there are some crucial differences.

Definition of restraint

The COP definition includes what is commonly referred to as chemical restraint (i.e., it covers the use of drugs, while the JCAHO restraint definition does not). The COP definition, however, is highly limited in that only drugs that are not a standard treatment for the patient's medical or psychiatric condition can be considered restraint. Note that the word *condition* and not *diagnosis* is used; therefore, if a patient is suffering from restlessness, lack of judgement, limited self-control, etc., regardless of diagnosis, these might well be considered as *conditions* that require treatment and for which there are standard treatments. The treatment might well include psychoactive drugs or sedatives.

The JCAHO's definition of restraint and restraint standards exclude *opt-outs* (see Chapter 1, p. 37 for more explanation of opt-outs). But the COP definition does not provide for any exclusions—there are no opt-outs. If strictly interpreted, this difference is likely to cause serious problems in medical and surgical settings. Specifically, the COP definition of restraint includes the following opt-outs that the JCAHO definition excludes: "immobilization related to medical, dental, diagnostic, or surgical procedures, etc.;" "adaptive support," "helmets," "therapeutic holding," and "forensic and correction restrictions ... for security purposes." This means that the COP considers as restraint the use of IV arm boards, papoose wraps for children undergoing minor surgery, and a host of similar procedures.

The COP definition does not make clear which standard applies to a patient who could be considered both medical and surgical and behavioral, while the JCAHO does have a clear distinction. For example, would a patient with a psychiatric diagnosis who is hospitalized for surgery and needs restraint be covered under the COP medical and surgical standard or the behavioral healthcare standard? The answer to this question is important because the medical and surgical and behavioral healthcare standards differ regarding the length of time for which a restraint order can be written.

Protocols

While the JCAHO permits properly trained and authorized nurses to use protocols to apply restraint without a doctor's order, the COP does not. The COP requires restraint to be used only after an order, and never after a standing order. The latter provision seems to rule out the use of a protocol even if a physician specifically orders use of a protocol for a particular patient. In addition, the COP does not mention emergency use of restraint in the absence of a physician. Nor does it deal with the issue of how long after issuing a telephone order a physician must see the patient face-to-face.

However, if, as seems likely, the COP guidelines do prohibit use of protocols, the JCAHO standards still do provide a method of achieving some of the benefit of using a protocol. JCAHO standard TX.7.5.3.1 gives a nurse who recognizes the need for restraint and initiates restraint 12 hours to notify the physician and get a telephone order. The physician then must examine the patient and write an order within 24 hours of the restraint initiation. In a medical and surgical setting, this approach eliminates the need for nurses to get a physician's order immediately for such common and relatively benign procedures as applying an arm board for a short period of time.

Involvement of the treating physician

The COP standard requires increased physician involvement in two aspects of restraint use in medical and surgical settings. In contrast, the thrust of the JCAHO's 1999 standards is to diminish physician involvement.

First, as mentioned above in regard to protocols, with its approval of nursing protocols and significant increase in the amount of time it allows a nurse to notify a physician after emergency use of restraint, the JCAHO has increased nursing authority and lightened the otherwise considerable load on physicians. The COP does not deal at all with emergency application of restraint in the absence of a physician—even though this is a relatively frequent event in hospitals. But it remains to be seen how strict HCFA will be in applying the new COP standards to this situation. Strict application would seem to be unworkable for many hospitals because of the need for immediate physician orders, when physicians are not always on the scene.

Second, the COP requires that when a physician who is not the treating physician writes an order for restraint, he or she must consult with the treating physician as soon as possible. (How "as soon as possible" will be interpreted is an important, and as yet unanswered, question.) JCAHO does not require this, although there are many who would say it should.

Modification of the care plan

The COP requires restraint use to be in accordance with "a written modification to the patient's plan of care." But the JCAHO does not require this, and it actually does not mention individual care plans at all in its restraint standards. In many instances, it is possible in the medical and surgical setting to anticipate the possible need for restraint and to write a care plan that provides for it before it is needed. In other cases, however, the care plan would have to be modified after restraint is applied. This is one additional paperwork item that hospitals must be concerned with.

Lacking 24-hour limit on orders

In contrast with the above items, in which the COP is more restrictive than the JCAHO standards, the COP does not limit the length of time for a restraint order, nor does it require that the order itself be time-limited, as the JCAHO standards do.

Lacking requirements for patient and family education or for performance improvement

Patient and family education and performance improvement are two more issues that the JCAHO considers important but that the COP does not deal with. The JCAHO lists patient and family education as a requirement in standard TX.7.1.1.4 and the intent of standard TX.7.5; and it requires performance improvement under standards TX.7.1.2 and TX.7.5.1.

Comparing the COP standards for "behavior management" with the JCAHO's hospital standards for behavioral healthcare patients

General comments

Many of the points above regarding the medical and surgical COP standard apply as well to the behavior management COP standard. They will not be repeated here in detail. These include the issues of chemical restraint, involvement of the treating physician, emergency use of restraint, time-limited orders, the care plan, patient and family education, and performance improvement.

Use of the term *behavior management* in the COP standard is different from the JCAHO's use of the term. The COP seems to intend that behavior management covers what the JCAHO calls behavioral health care and more (see below).

Definitions of restraint *and* seclusion

The discussion above regarding the difference between the COP medical and surgical standard's definition of restraint and the JCAHO's definition also applies to the behavior management standard's definition of restraint. There is a difference as well between the COP definition of seclusion and that of the JCAHO. The JCAHO specifies that seclusion requires the patient to be alone in the room, while the COP does not mention this. The COP definition includes in its definition of seclusion a situation in which a staff observer is in the seclusion room with the patient. The COP definition seems to be more realistic than the JCAHO's definition, since seclusion is occasionally carried out with a staff observer in the seclusion room, but the basic seclusion process is still being applied.

Quite commonly, restraint in behavioral healthcare settings is carried out in a room in which the patient is alone. For some patients, restraint is more calming when the patient is alone and is observed only from outside the room. JCAHO surveyors have always treated this situation simply as restraint. The COP, in contrast, deals separately with restraint and seclusion "used simultaneously" and restraint. Many hospitals are likely to miss this distinction and assume they are using restraint alone, when in the classification of the COP, they are using restraint and seclusion simultaneously. The COP states specific monitoring requirements for restraint and seclusion used simultaneously—either face-to-face or both video and audio by an "assigned" staff member. However, the COP requires continual assessment and monitoring for all patients in restraint or seclusion, so there appears to be a distinction without a difference.

Restraint or seclusion as part of a behavior management plan

For several years, the JCAHO has had a number of standards relating to behavior management procedures. The JCAHO defines behavior management as, among other things, "using basic learning techniques." Although the COP does not define precisely what it means by behavior management, the context in which the term is used implies that it deals with behavior associated with mental illness and similar disorder, such as intoxication.

Thus the COP's definition of behavior management is much broader than the JCAHO's. Even more significant, the COP behavior management standard seems to be even more broadly applicable than the JCAHO restraint standards for behavioral healthcare patients. The JCAHO standards are limited in applicability to patients in behavioral health (i.e., psychiatric) units in acute care hospitals and to freestanding psychiatric hospitals. The JCAHO standards do not cover patients in non-behavioral settings (e.g., the emergency department or a medical/surgical unit) who need to be restrained for apparently behavioral reasons, whereas the COP standards do. As discussed above, in practice this means that the COP standard applies, for example, to a mentally ill patient restrained in a medical and surgical unit.

Sometimes, what we refer to elsewhere as *contingent restraint* or *seclusion* is used as part of a behavior management program. In dealing with extremely explosive and potentially dangerous patients, some organizations have found that restraint or seclusion can be effective negative reinforcers. To apply restraint and seclusion for this purpose, however, organizations must outline the criteria for applying the restraint or seclusion (i.e., which behaviors trigger the use of restraint or seclusion) in the behavior management plan *before* the need for restraint or seclusion. The JCAHO requires a behavior management program to be designed by a qualified mental health professional (commonly a Ph.D. psychologist with relevant specialty training) but otherwise permits its use. The plan can provide for initiation of restraint or seclusion without a doctor's order each time. The COP does not permit restraint and seclusion as part of a behavior management program unless a doctor orders restraint or seclusion before each use, and restricts the use of restraint or seclusion only to emergency situations, in any case.

Physician face-to-face evaluation within one hour of restraint

Currently, in most behavioral healthcare settings, when nurses recognize the emergency need for restraint or seclusion, they use the indicated process and then immediately call for a physician's order (in compliance with JCAHO standards). If the physician is not immediately available to see the patient, he or she issues a telephone order that then can be extended in increments for up to 24 hours. The physician is not required to examine the patient unless he or she wishes to renew the order beyond 24 hours. This approach is particularly useful in smaller hospitals, in which relatively few or no physicians are available, and it is troublesome to disturb physicians during office hours or in the middle of the night.

The new COP rules out this approach. Although telephone orders are still acceptable in an emergency, the physician must see the patient within one hour. Obviously, this is going to require waking physicians in the middle of the night or disturbing them during other activities and getting them to come to the hospital promptly.

Patients restrained by medication: assessment, monitoring, evaluation

Unlike the JCAHO, which does not deal with "chemical restraint," the COP includes under its definition of restraint the use of medication intended to restrain patients. The significant impact of this is that chemically restrained patients will have to be assessed, monitored, and evaluated in exactly the same way in which mechanically restrained patients are. Orders for restraint via medication will have to meet the requirements for restraint orders (i.e., the patient must be seen within one hour, the order is good for no longer than four hours for adults, unless extended, and in any case for no more than 24 hours, etc.). This represents a considerable increase in staff time and paperwork requirements.

Death reporting

The COP requires that restraint- and seclusion-related deaths must be reported to HCFA. What is not clear is whether the report must include the patient's name and the details of the occurrence or simply the fact that a death has occurred. The degree of confidentiality protection, if any, either type of report would receive is also unclear. At present, JCAHO-accredited facilities are required to report sentinel events to JCAHO—which includes restraint- and seclusion-related deaths—but there are significant confidentiality protections, with more presumably on the way.

Note: Figure B, p.17, provides a summary of the main issues on which the COP requirements go beyond those of the JCAHO

Figure A **New COP Restraint Standards for Hospitals**

Note: The following text is directly excerpted from The Federal Register, July 2, 1999, Volume 64, Number 127.

Sec.482.13 (e) Standard: Restraint for acute medical and surgical care.

(1) The patient has the right to be free from restraints of any form that are not medically necessary or are used as a means of coercion, discipline, convenience, or retaliation by staff. The term "restraint" includes either a physical restraint or a drug that is being used as a restraint. A physical restraint is any manual method or physical or mechanical device, material, or equipment attached or adjacent to the patient's body that he or she cannot easily remove that restricts freedom of movement or normal access to one's body. A drug used as a restraint is a medication used to control behavior or to restrict the patient's freedom of movement and is not a standard treatment for the patient's medical or psychiatric condition.

(2) A restraint can only be used if needed to improve the patient's well-being and less restrictive interventions have been determined to be ineffective.

(3) The use of a restraint must be—

- (i) Selected only when other less restrictive measures have been found to be ineffective to protect the patient or others from harm;
- (ii) In accordance with the order of a physician or other licensed independent practitioner permitted by the State and hospital to order a restraint. This order must—
  - (A) Never be written as a standing or on an as needed basis (that is, PRN); and
  - (B) Be followed by a consultation with the patient's treating physician, as soon as possible, if the restraint is not ordered by the patient's treating physician;
- (iii) In accordance with a written modification to the patient's plan of care;
- (iv) Implemented in the least restrictive manner possible;
- (v) In accordance with safe and appropriate restraining techniques; and
- (vi) Ended at the earliest possible time.

(4) The condition of the restrained patient must be continually assessed, monitored, and reevaluated.

Figure A **New COP Restraint Standards for Hospitals (cont.)**

(5) All staff who have direct patient contact must have ongoing education and training in the proper and safe use of restraints.

(f) Standard: Seclusion and Restraint for behavior management.

(1) The patient has the right to be free from seclusion and restraints, of any form, imposed as a means of coercion, discipline, convenience, or retaliation by staff. The term "restraint" includes either a physical restraint or a drug that is being used as a restraint. A physical restraint is any manual method or physical or mechanical device, material, or equipment attached or adjacent to the patient's body that he or she cannot easily remove that restricts freedom of movement or normal access to one's body. A drug used as a restraint is a medication used to control behavior or to restrict the patient's freedom of movement and is not a standard treatment for the patient's medical or psychiatric condition. Seclusion is the involuntary confinement of a person in a room or an area where the person is physically prevented from leaving.

(2) Seclusion or a restraint can only be used in emergency situations if needed to ensure the patient's physical safety and less restrictive interventions have been determined to be ineffective.

(3) The use of a restraint or seclusion must be—

- (i) Selected only when less restrictive measures have been found to be ineffective to protect the patient or others from harm:
- (ii) In accordance with the order of a physician or other licensed independent practitioner permitted by the State and the hospital to order seclusion or restraint. The following requirements will be superseded by existing State laws that are more restrictive:
  - (A) Orders for the use of seclusion or a restraint must never be written as a standing order or on an as needed basis (that is, PRN).
  - (B) The treating physician must be consulted as soon as possible if the restraint or seclusion is not ordered by the patient's treating physician.

Figure A **New COP Restraint Standards for Hospitals (cont.)**

(C) A physician or other licensed independent practitioner must see and evaluate the need for restraint or seclusion within 1 hour after the initiation of this intervention.

(D) Each written order for a physical restraint or seclusion is limited to 4 hours for adults; 2 hours for children and adolescents ages 9 to 17; or 1 hour for patients under 9. The original order may only be renewed in accordance with these limits for up to a total of 24 hours. After the original order expires, a physician or licensed independent practitioner (if allowed under State law) must see and assess the patient before issuing a new order.

(iii) In accordance with a written modification to the patient's plan of care;

(iv) Implemented in the least restrictive manner possible;

(v) In accordance with safe appropriate restraining techniques; and

(vi) Ended at the earliest possible time.

(4) A restraint and seclusion may not be used simultaneously unless the patient is—

(i) Continually monitored face-to-face by an assigned staff member; or

(ii) Continually monitored by staff using both video and audio equipment. This monitoring must be in close proximity to the patient.

(5) The condition of the patient who is in a restraint or in seclusion must continually be assessed, monitored, and reevaluated.

(6) All staff who have direct patient contact must have ongoing education and training in the proper and safe use of seclusion and restraint application and techniques and alternative methods for handling behavior, symptoms, and situations that traditionally have been treated through the use of restraints or seclusion.

(7) The hospital must report to HCFA any death that occurs while a patient is restrained or in seclusion, or where it is reasonable to assume that a patient's death is a result of restraint or seclusion.

Figure B

Issues on which the Conditions of Participation go beyond the JCAHO Standards

Keep an eye on the following issues on which the Conditions of Participation go beyond the JCAHO requirements.

Issue	COP Requirement
Chemical restraint	Use of drugs as restraint must be handled exactly the same as physical restraint (e.g., orders, time limits, monitoring, documentation etc.)
Inclusive definition of restraint	There are no exclusions for such purposes as medical immobilization or postural support
Nursing protocols eliminated	There can be no use of restraint without a doctor's order
Consultation with treating physician	Restraint by order of a physician who is not the "treating physician" must be followed as soon as possible by consultation with the treating physician
Amended care plan	The care plan must provide for restraint, so unexpected use of restraint requires changing the care plan
Behavior management	COP definition is broad, but not precise, while JCAHO definition is narrow; COP rules out use of restraint or seclusion as part of a behavior management program (i.e., as negative reinforcer)
Face-to-face assessment	In behavior management (what JCAHO calls behavioral health care plus other related circumstances), a telephone order for restraint or seclusion must be followed within one hour by a doctor's face-to-face patient assessment
Observation process	In behavior management, a restrained patient alone in a room must be "continually" monitored either face-to-face or by video and audio
Death reporting	In behavior management, all restraint- and seclusion-related deaths must be reported to HCFA

Introduction

Lessons Learned about Restraint since 1996

Restraint and seclusion have been the subject of intense scrutiny and debate in healthcare organizations striving to gain JCAHO accreditation since the inception of the 1996 restraint and seclusion standards. As an expert on restraint- and seclusion-related issues, both before and after 1996, I have observed numerous episodes of restraint and seclusion in a variety of healthcare settings, interviewed clinical personnel who were involved with restraint, and spoken with patients who were restrained. As a result of these experiences, but with no claim to any type of systematic study, I believe it is imperative that any organization seeking to improve its restraint and seclusion policies and practice pay specific attention to the following issues.

Restraint is dangerous and demeaning to patients

Although the first edition of this book made the point, my experience in the last few years suggests the point needs repeating: Restraint is dangerous. There are no comprehensive national statistics on deaths associated with restraint, but several studies have attempted to count the cases. Based on these studies, it is safe to estimate that in the last four or five years there were several hundred such deaths in psychiatric facilities and perhaps an equal number in acute care and long-term care facilities. There is less information on the frequency of restraint use than for restraint-related deaths, but some facilities are now counting episodes and tracking frequency statistics. These statistics are valuable because they can show patterns and trends in restraint-related injuries and deaths, which is the first step in preventing them.

Stories and reports from people who have been restrained (either for behavioral or for medical or surgical reasons) all end with the same conclusion: Restraint is, at best, a discomfiting and traumatic experience. I have never encountered a patient who was grateful for having been restrained or who reported that it was a positive experience, although I recognize that such patients might exist. On the other hand, I have heard from and read about many patients who state that restraint was a terrible experience and was not justified. I do not assume that all these patients are able to accurately judge or report what happened to them. Yet the overwhelming consensus makes a strong case against the debilitating aspects of restraint and seclusion. (See Chapter 3 for more discussion regarding negative effects of restraint and seclusion.)

My personal opinion on the use of restraint or seclusion remains what it has been over the past several years: Restraint or seclusion can be compared to open-heart surgery—it is probably a life-saving procedure in the rare instances it is absolutely needed. Restraint or seclusion should never be used when there is doubt about whether it is needed. And when it is needed, it should never be undertaken lightly and should always be considered a high-risk procedure that can have disastrous effects.

Restraint use in medical and surgical settings still tends to be ignored

The determination of whether a procedure is actually restraint—and the JCAHO restraint standards apply—or whether it is a restraint-like procedure that can be considered an "opt-out" not covered by the JCAHO standards remains unclear. The JCAHO has not made a major effort to clarify its definition of restraint and essentially leaves it up to individual organizations to develop their own definitions. The problem this presents is that some hospitals tie up patients fairly often, but do not consider this to be restraint. In reality, however, this tying up (1) appears to be restraint to outside observers, (2) feels like restraint to patients, and (3) usually presents the same dangers and negative effects as restraint. Chapter 1, p. 37, discusses this issue in greater detail.

Documentation is important and needs improvement

Every episode of restraint or seclusion should be extensively documented, primarily in the patient's record. (Some organizations also document it in a specific restraint log.) Documentation is one of an organization's best protections against unjust accusations of improper restraint use and is also an important base for quality improvement efforts. But documentation remains inconsistent and incomplete in many facilities, thus exposing organizations to noncompliance scores from the JCAHO and to liability lawsuits.

Many clinical personnel do not realize the importance of clear and complete documentation. They need to be frequently reminded that clinical records exist not only for the use of those caring for the patient or even just for staff working in the facility—records also can be used as evidence in a lawsuit and even as material to be published in the newspaper. Hostile parties, such as a plaintiff's attorney, can minutely dissect medical records.

Chronic problem areas that need improvement so clinical records can hold up under critical and intense scrutiny include the following:

- All entries in clinical records should not only be dated but should also have an accurate time. Physicians in particular commonly fail to note the time. If the organization's policy on documentation requires noting the time, failure to do so is a clear instance of noncompliance with the JCAHO standards. Regardless of organizational policy, however, the absence of time on a record or order can make it impossible to demonstrate that actions were performed in accordance with other policy requirements, JCAHO standards, and most importantly, good clinical care.

- Clinical justification for using restraint or seclusion is often poorly described or not described at all. Personnel in many facilities routinely write "danger to self or others" in orders or progress notes as a justification with no further explanation. Some facilities even use preprinted checklists with a box or two that can be checked to indicate "danger to self or others" and does not even leave space to expand or elaborate. Good documentation of clinical justification includes a description of the patient's behavior, the less restrictive alternatives to restraint or seclusion that were unsuccessfully tried, and the education efforts, if any, attempted prior to or at the time of application of restraint. (In an emergency, documentation can be completed after the application of restraint, but before key personnel leave the clinical unit.) (See Chapter 4 for more discussion of clinical justification and related documentation.)

- Use of verbal/telephone orders and the documentation of these orders are frequently not done properly. The most common problem areas are:
  - countersignatures are not dated and not timed;
  - physicians do not write a note to demonstrate their knowledge of the situation, agreement with the action, and current assessment of the patient when they countersign the order; and
  - aspects of the documentation are inconsistent and possibly false, as when one part of the record implies that restraint was applied before the order was received, while another part describes the order as coming first.

The JCAHO requires that only authorized personnel can receive telephone orders (telephone orders are even more of a problem than verbal orders). Organizations should always require recording the date, time, name of person issuing the order, and name of person receiving the order for all verbal and telephone orders. Many organizations (and some states) also require that the order be authenticated or countersigned by whomever issued the order, usually within 24 hours (the JCAHO no longer requires this).

Physician involvement needs more emphasis

One of the most important groups—certainly, in some facilities, the most important group—in determining restraint and seclusion use is physicians. Physicians are ultimately responsible for all aspects of treatment of their patients.

Paradoxically, physicians seem to receive little or no training on using restraint and seclusion as part of the treatment process, and they often know little about it. Organizations appear to presume that physicians will somehow intuitively know the advantages and disadvantages of restraint and seclusion use and will know when restraint or seclusion is appropriate. In reality, as we have come to know more about the effects of restraint and seclusion, we have come to recognize that the decision to use these procedures is quite complex and requires weighing a number of pros and cons. Appropriate decision making requires a good deal of information.

Organizations should train physicians on restraint and seclusion use. Training should include information regarding the following:

- indications and contraindications for use;
- the risks and concerns regarding restraint use;
- use of less restrictive alternatives;
- assessment of patients before issuing an initial restraint order and at the point of renewal of the order;
- appropriate documentation techniques;
- national standards, state laws and regulations, and local policies; and
- methods of applying and removing restraint.

In addition, when possible, training should include observation of restrained or secluded patients, interviewing of patients who have been restrained or secluded, and brief personal experience in restraint or seclusion.

Contrary to good clinical practice and JCAHO expectations, some facilities view restraint or seclusion as purely a nursing staff issue. In these cases, the physician's role is to ratify the decision nurses made, sometimes long after nurses made the decision to initiate restraint. Uninvolved or absentee physicians leave themselves and their institutions open to serious criticism. Although nurses are empowered to deal with serious emergencies in the absence of the physician, the expectation is that they will notify the physician about what happened and receive further direction as soon as possible. In addition, physicians should plan in advance to use less restrictive alternatives to restraint that are specific to each patient. Physicians should also document their own involvement through notes in treatment plans and/or progress notes.

Healthcare organizations should direct measures aimed at reducing the frequency of restraint use to both physicians and nurses, since the frequency of its use depends in no small part on physician decisions (or nursing decisions then ratified by physicians).

Therapeutic holding needs clarification

The meaning of the term *therapeutic holding* varies from organization to organization, and therefore, the applicability of JCAHO standards to it is unclear. What is clear is that whenever staff use physical force against patients—which is always an element in therapeutic holding—the danger of injury to patients, staff, or both is high. A large proportion of restraint-related deaths occur either during therapeutic holding or shortly after. (Chapter 2 discusses therapeutic holding in detail.)

The major questions and issues surrounding therapeutic holding include the following:

- *Is staff grappling with a patient ever "therapeutic" (i.e., part of the treatment)? If so, do the positive aspects ever outweigh the dangers?* There is no evidence-based answer to this question. Some theorists suggest that physical restraint (i.e., therapeutic holding) is more beneficial than mechanical restraint (i.e., restraining via devices). They argue that physical restraint communicates positive emotion and concern while mechanical restraint communicates rejection and abandonment, particularly with children. However, others have postulated the theory that for those patients who have been physically abused, holding can reactivate traumatic memories and make the situation worse. Whether therapeutic holding is as dangerous or more dangerous than use of mechanical restraints, good clinical care suggests that holding be regulated and monitored as if it were restraint.

- *Is therapeutic holding considered to be restraint, and therefore covered by JCAHO standards?* Different JCAHO officials have given different answers to this question. The introduction to the restraint and seclusion standards does not definitively state if the restraint and seclusion standards apply to therapeutic holding.

- *Is therapeutic holding (other than as an emergency measure until mechanical restraints can be applied) ever acceptable with patients older than seven or eight years?* Clearly the risk of injury increases as the size and strength of the patient increases. Furthermore, with some patients, the prolonged use of direct person-to-person force invites resistance, struggle, and possibly escalation in violence. The result is an intensification of the patient's excitement rather than a de-escalation of it, and staff might even lose control of the situation due to their own exhaustion or anger. Anecdotal reports suggest that some staff, when they engage in an intense struggle with a patient, resort to maneuvers that are appropriate for a wrestling match but are not acceptable in clinical care.

Use of advance directives as a way of reducing psychological trauma

Advance directives relating to end-of-life care have become a common concern in hospitals since the passage of the federal Patient Self Determination Act. Regarding restraint and seclusion, advance directives have a different focus. Many psychiatric patients wish to determine in advance whether restraint or seclusion will be used on them. According to patients and patient advocates, just by giving patients a choice—even if sometimes the choice cannot be followed because of clinical circumstances—healthcare professionals strengthen the therapeutic relationship, facilitate recovery, and reduce the psychological trauma of restraint and seclusion. (Chapter 3, p.63, discusses this issue further.)

Patient and family education is commonly neglected

JCAHO standards require that staff educate patients—and their families, provided that staff have the patient's consent or the consent of the patient's guardian—regarding the use of restraint or seclusion. Some psychiatric facilities meet this requirement effectively and easily by preparing a brochure on restraint that they distribute to all patients and their families upon admission. Such brochures state that occasionally staff must resort to restraint and that any patient might encounter another patient being restrained. The brochures go on to explain the reasons for the process and how it is carried out.

Most facilities, however, do not fulfill this requirement in any meaningful way at all. (Because JCAHO surveyors are influenced by consensus and common practice, the relevant Patient and Family Education standard is rarely scored as noncompliant even though it should be, if strictly interpreted.) The most common way of dealing with the standard is to tell patients—only after they have been placed in restraint or seclusion—what they did to precipitate it and what they have to do to get released. This is essential information, but it does not go far enough. The other patients need to know what is going on, lest they be frightened or upset. Family members need to know what is happening to their loved one and why (always with the patient's consent). Patients are probably too upset at the time of application of restraint or seclusion to absorb much of what they are told.

Educating patients about restraint before the need for restraint even exists is the best clinical practice, especially in acute care facilities, in which there are few formal efforts to meet this requirement. When patients are restrained in the course of medical or surgical treatment, no doubt they are told what is happening as part of good nursing care, but education in advance of the treatment is preferable. (See Chapter 4 for more on patient and family education.)

Restraint and seclusion are sometimes inappropriately used as punishment

Almost all healthcare professionals are aware that for a number of reasons it is absolutely unacceptable to use restraint or seclusion as punishment. (As discussed in Chapter 2, one exception is "contingent" restraint or seclusion used as part of an individually designed behavior management program.) But the line between emergency use of restraint or seclusion to control a dangerously violent patient and use of restraint or seclusion to teach the patient not to behave that way again (i.e., punishment) after the violence has subsided is often unclear. As Chapter 2, p. 51, discusses further, it is important that appropriate consideration and staff training on this issue is critical.

Staff training and competency evaluation are often poorly done

Obviously, a well-trained, conscientious, and caring staff is key to the advantageous and proper use of restraint. In reality, most facilities consider only very limited aspects of the overall training that is necessary. The most common form of training such facilities offer is limited to short presentations regarding the psychological aspects of conflict resolution or anger management, de-escalation, and some hands-on practice applying restraints. This training is usually required for all clinical personnel, excluding physicians, and is usually offered either during an initial orientation period or as part of required annual training.

Although surveyors rarely expect any training beyond that described above, such training is far from sufficient for clinical personnel. Although front-line staff need to know how to de-escalate tense situations and, when that fails, how to get a resisting patient under physical control, many other skills are also needed, particularly for higher-level personnel. (See Chapter 4, Figure 4.2, for more information.) In particular,

- Nurses need training to recognize when emergency application of restraint is appropriate since they have the authority under JCAHO standards and state laws to initiate emergency restraint use. The skills required for emergency restraint application include a rapid assessment of two major factors: (1) the availability and likely effectiveness of alternatives to restraint, and (2) the patient's physical and mental ability to withstand the stresses of restraint.

- Nurses need training in supervising the actual application of restraint. Typically, nurses receive the same training as all other clinical personnel in de-escalation and restraint application. But when a patient requires restraint, it is usually the senior nurse who directs the process. Effective teamwork is critical to avoid distress and injury; good leadership can make the difference to this end.

- Nurses and other staff who monitor restrained patients need training in how to observe patients and how to document the care appropriately. They need to be knowledgeable about the criteria for removing a patient from restraint or seclusion, and also about the indications that the patient is suffering physical or mental distress, which requires restraint removal.

- Nurses or other "licensed, qualified, and authorized" individuals in behavioral healthcare settings who have authority to extend the duration of restraint or seclusion orders repeatedly up to 24 hours need training in the requisite face-to-face assessments for such extensions. This assessment should focus on the need to continue the restraint versus factors for discontinuation; alternatives to restraint; and how restraint or seclusion relates to the patient's treatment plan. Documentation of this assessment must be thorough enough to demonstrate that the assessment was conducted properly.

- Finally, organizations should consider what training is necessary for physicians and any other licensed independent practitioners authorized to order restraint. The JCAHO does not require any training for these individuals, but as discussed earlier in this section, training is critical for physicians (see p. 22).

More attention to the use of alternatives to restraint or seclusion is needed

Alternatives to restraint fall into two categories: (1) those that have to be carried out long in advance of the patient's crisis and (2) those that are carried out concurrently with the crisis to try to end it.

The first group of alternatives generally applies to the patient group as a whole. For example, clinical experience suggests that patients are more likely to lose control in crowded living conditions, in which there is no opportunity to be alone, little opportunity for vigorous activity, and limited interaction with staff.

Clinical experience also suggests that the "culture" of the patient group—the tone and generally accepted forms of behavior among patients—strongly influences what patients will do when they are upset. Crowded living conditions and group culture are not situations that the JCAHO requires organizations to alter before the application of restraint or seclusion, but they are nevertheless important and must be considered before patients even arrive at the facility. The decision to consider these factors in relation to reducing the frequency of restraint is usually an administrative one, and the value of these factors in reducing the need for restraint is often underappreciated.

The second group of restraint alternatives focuses on the individual patient. These include traditional techniques such as de-escalation, distraction, and medication use. In too many situations, staff are not sensitive to the buildup of tension in one or more patients and therefore do not act until there is an explosion.

Determining which alternative to use—and when—is a complex decision, requiring a good deal of training. Documentation in clinical records should reveal that alternatives to restraint were attempted before restraint was used. In some facilities, staff use checklists to indicate which alternatives were tried unsuccessfully. The danger with this approach is that the documentation can be generic and vague, and checklists do not require staff to make a genuine effort to see if any alternatives will work.

JCAHO surveyors and central office staff sometimes interpret standards differently

The JCAHO has made major efforts in recent years to make the standards easier to understand and apply. Specifically, the standards have been rewritten in simple language, and many standards contain supplemental intent statements that provide additional clarification and examples of compliance that provide concrete—but not binding—advice. Before new standards take effect, they are field-tested by a variety of clinicians and administrators, sometimes through mock surveys.

Despite these efforts, occasionally standards are not clear or might even be confusing. In these instances, organizations are free to consult the Standards Interpretation Unit at the JCAHO for a ruling. Surveyors might also make an interpretive ruling during a survey. But regarding restraint, such rulings are not always consistent. Inconsistency produces confusion, which makes it difficult to properly prepare for a survey and is a possible risk-management issue. When rulings are inconsistent, organizations risk being scored as noncompliant even though they are doing what they have been advised to do by someone at the JCAHO.

Some of the standards that produce the most confusion include those relating to

- the definition and limits on the use of therapeutic holding;
- the limits of "opt-outs" (those practices that might involve the use of restraining devices but that the JCAHO excludes from its restraint standards);
- the permissibility of restraint use without physician orders as part of a formal behavior management program; and
- the definition of a *restraint episode*.

There are two steps to take to deal with the problem of inconsistent interpretations. First, when an organization obtains an interpretation of a standard from someone speaking on behalf of the JCAHO, it should obtain that interpretation in writing. Second, regardless of what the JCAHO interpretation is, organizations should provide what they consider to be good clinical care. This might not always be consistent with what the standards seem to require. One example of this is the use of opt-outs: good clinical care means they should be treated as restraint, although JCAHO standards do not require it.

Reducing restraint use requires an attitude adjustment

Over the country, there are amazing variations in the manner and frequency of restraint use from organization to organization, even when those organizations serve exactly the same sort of patients. Some facilities have managed to reduce restraint use by 50% to 75% or more in the space of a few years without any increase in injuries to patients or staff from out-of-control patients. What can explain this dramatic reduction?

The obvious explanation is a change in the way these facilities address violence-prone patients and the general atmosphere of the patient care setting. Some organizations spend great effort training staff to use restraint alternatives and facilitate their use. Others do not. Some organizations have settings that discourage violence, while others lend themselves to loss of control over situations. In some organizations, every episode of restraint is viewed as a treatment failure—even if only a minor one—while in other organizations, restraint use is considered a routine event, similar to dispensing medications.

The implication is that organizations can change the way restraint is used to improve patient safety and patient care. This is not an easy task because there are few things as difficult to change as patient and staff culture and customs (however, altering the physical environment on a limited budget might be just as difficult). Certainly, the first steps involve improving policies and providing training. But these are only the first steps. The critical challenge is revising deep-seated attitudes and habits.

Chapter One

Defining Restraint and Seclusion

An appropriate, clear definition of restraint is important

Restraint use is potentially dangerous both to restrained patients and to staff members who must apply restraint to resistant patients. Therefore, various legal restrictions and regulatory and accreditation standards apply to each use—or *episode*—of restraint in an effort to minimize the risk of injury or harm. Failure to comply with these restrictions or standards can result in serious consequences for an organization, such as injury to patients or staff members or legal and regulatory penalties. For these reasons, it is imperative that anyone using or supervising restraint knows its potential dangers, alternative strategies, and relevant standards and regulations.

But those who use and supervise restraint might ask: "When do these standards and regulations apply?" and "Which devices and procedures fall under the definition of restraint?" Surprisingly, these are not simple questions with simple answers. Official definitions of restraint vary, depending upon the organization defining it and the type of organization in which restraint is being used. Furthermore, application of the Joint Commission on Accreditation of Healthcare Organizations' (JCAHO) definition, which is most relevant to this discussion, is partially subjective—and therefore not always clear—because it revolves around the interpretation of the intent of those who use restraint (see p. 37 for more discussion).

The Health Care Financing Administration's definition

The most inclusive definition of restraint is the one that the federal government applies in long-term care facilities. This definition—provided in both the Health Care Financing Administration's (HCFA) Interpretive Guidelines to the Omnibus

Reconciliation Act (OBRA) of 1987 and the February 6, 1992, Federal Register (v. 57, no. 24, paragraph 483.13[a][1][i])—describes physical restraint as follows:

> *Physical restraint: Any manual method or physical or mechanical device, material, or equipment attached or adjacent to the resident's body that the resident cannot remove easily, which restricts freedom of movement or access to his or her body. Physical restraints include leg restraints, arm restraints, hand mitts, soft ties or vests, and wheelchair safety bars.*

HCFA's definition is relatively objective. There is little room for confusion or misunderstanding because the definition clearly encompasses every sort of physical restriction on a patient's movement. Therefore, the federal government's regulations regarding restraint apply to everything that could possibly be considered restraint. (Note: This definition and accompanying regulations apply only to long-term care; not to acute care hospitals and other types of facilities. As of August 1, 1999, however, a federal definition of restraint has gone into effect in hospitals [see *New in 1999: Federal Standards on Restraint and Seclusion in Hospitals*, p. 1 for more discussion].)

Healthcare organizations other than long-term care facilities are not required (and usually cannot afford) to apply this definition of restraint because it is too broad for practical purposes. Organizations do not have the time or resources to complete the requisite documentation in every instance in which a procedure fits the above definition. The difficulty, therefore, is creating a definition for organizations that corresponds with the best clinical practice and ensures patient safety but doesn't unduly burden organizations with paperwork.

The JCAHO's definition of restraint

The JCAHO has struggled over the past several years to define and limit the use of restraint. The most recent JCAHO definition, which took effect July 1, 1996, and which presumably supersedes the prior definition, is not a single clear statement but is contained in several statements.

The following selected excerpts, from pages TX–47 and TX–48 of the *1999 Comprehensive Accreditation Manual for Hospitals (CAMH)*, describe the JCAHO's current view of restraint:

> *In its broadest context, restraint is any method of physically restricting a person's freedom of movement, physical activity, or normal access to his or her body. In the context of these standards, restraint is considered involuntary use either as part of an approved protocol, or as indicated by individual orders.*
>
> *The standards do not apply to*
>
> - *standard practices that include temporary immobilization or limitation of mobility related to medical, dental, diagnostic, or surgical procedures and the related post-procedure care processes (for example, surgical positioning, IV arm boards, radiotherapy procedures, protection of surgical and treatment sites in pediatric patients); or*
>
> - *adaptive support in response to assessed patient need (for example, postural support, orthopedic appliances, or tabletop chairs).*

The overall thrust of the JCAHO's current definition of restraint is to encourage the reduction of its use and encourage alternative interventions. The flexibility of the definition also allows organizations and restraint users to determine for themselves whether a particular procedure or device constitutes restraint. It is less prescriptive than in the past and permits individual organizations to establish practices, policies, and procedures that meet their unique needs. Therefore, a hospital's own restraint definition, as outlined in its policies, preempts the JCAHO definition, provided it is not less restrictive than the JCAHO's.

Your definition of restraint

As noted above, the JCAHO allows healthcare organizations to develop and use a definition of restraint that best fits their individual needs and practices. We recommend that an organization define restraint broadly—encompassing all procedures that can reasonably be considered restraint. Hospitals can benefit from considering many procedures and situations that are commonly excluded from definitions of restraint as restraint because those situations usually carry the same risk of danger and negative effects as restraint. For example, a hospital might elect to consider all use of bedside rails as restraint, even though the JCAHO does not require it.

On the other hand, there are situations that hospitals can decide to exclude from their restraint definitions, such as use of arm boards to protect intravenous lines. In such instances, although staff should handle the procedure with the same observation and protective measures as they would with restraint, they are not required to complete extensive paperwork that restraint and other high-risk procedures demand.

Our recommendation for a broad definition of restraint is also intended to emphasize that, when in doubt, an organization should treat any procedure that might possibly be considered restraint as restraint. For instance, if an organization uses a device for some reason other than restraint, but there is a chance an outside observer (such as a surveyor) might consider it restraint, the burden is on the organization to demonstrate that restraint is not being used. For example, a Posey vest used to tie a patient into a chair could be postural support or restraint. Hospitals can best resolve such questions by creating a policy—approved by the medical staff—that clearly establishes the border between restraint use and other procedures.

Educating staff about the definition of restraint

Healthcare organizations need to educate staff about the definition of restraint because many professionals still incorrectly think of restraint in very narrow terms. They limit restraint to the application of leather cuffs to a psychiatric patient's limbs to tie the patient into bed (usually referred to as *four-point restraint* or *five-point restraint* when a fifth tie around the patient's waist, chest, or neck is included). These professionals do not consider other kinds of ties or physical restrictions—such as straps on a gurney or stretcher, mitts covering the hands to prevent scratching, or ties on both hands when an IV is running—as restraint.

This misunderstanding leads many hospital staff members to perpetuate the mistaken belief that they do not use restraint and that restraint use is limited to psychiatric hospitals. In reality, however, an acute care hospital that does not use restraint as part of patient care (within any reasonable or accepted definition of restraint) is extremely rare, if one exists at all. Therefore, the first step in reducing restraint frequency is to broaden staffs' understanding of what does and does not constitute restraint and to train them accordingly.

Situations in which "opt-outs" apply

Not every restriction on a patient's movement need be considered restraint, according to the JCAHO definition. Some devices, materials, and techniques that restrict patients' movements are often, if not always, used for purposes other than restraint, such as

- devices used for postural support, such as when staff use a cushion to support a sitting patient who is too weak to sit unaided, or use a Posey vest to keep a patient from falling out of a chair;
- devices used as regular, necessary aspects of certain procedures and treatments for medical immobilization, such as a mechanical device to position and hold a patient's body during a surgical procedure;
- mechanisms that improve a patient's ability to function or prevent further accidental injury, such as plaster casts, bandages, cervical collars, and limb braces;
- devices that prevent patients with cognitive deficits from unintentionally harming themselves, such as bed rails, helmets, and halter-type devices that prevent patients from falling out of bed; and
- devices applied for some other purpose that secondarily restrict patients—such as mittens used to apply medication to hands, or supports used during x-rays.

We call this group of procedures *opt-outs*. The JCAHO excludes opt-outs from its definition of restraint in its hospital, ambulatory care, and behavioral healthcare accreditation manuals, even though opt-outs restrict patient movement. The factor that determines whether such devices are considered restraint (at least as far as the JCAHO is concerned) is the intention of the person applying the device—not the device characteristics. This is why the JCAHO definition is partially subjective and murky. How can an observer be sure that what a user later reports as the intention of the application of a device is accurate—particularly when so much of the accreditation score depends on whether the user complied with standards when he or she applied restraint?

Hospitals must be aware of the difference between the JCAHO's definition of opt-outs and its definition of restraint when they attempt to classify as an opt-out an episode that could be considered restraint. Using opt-outs can make paperwork easier, although using opt-outs should never tempt an organization to relax its vigilance in protecting patients from the harmful effects of restraint or restraint-like activities. We again emphasize that even if the JCAHO does not consider a procedure restraint, it is often good clinical practice to indicate that the restrictions, observation requirements, documentation requirements, and physician orders required for restraint apply to the procedure. (Figure 1.1 summarizes situations that constitute restraint and fall under the JCAHO standards and requisite follow-up actions.)

Opt-outs and unconscious patients

Although unconscious patients are almost always protected by some sort of safety device, such as bed rails (some unconscious patients move vigorously and are protected by devices that are even more restrictive than bed rails), a hospital does not need to consider the use of such devices on unconscious patients as restraint, unless it chooses to do so or unless state regulations require it. (Even in these opt-out situations, however, nursing staff often monitor unconscious patients beyond the extent required for restrained patients because of the underlying conditions that cause the unconsciousness.)

Opt-outs and consent

The JCAHO considers voluntary consent to restraint an opt-out as well. Consent does not even need to be in writing—although written consent still serves as the best evidence of consent. The concept of implied consent—when a patient is not asked for and does not give written consent, but obviously cooperates with a procedure—is well recognized in medicine.

Figure 1.1 **Levels of Restraint Use and Their Applicability to the JCAHO Standards**

Type of Restraint or Seclusion	Do Standards Apply?	Required Actions
Level 1: Associated with standard practice for medical, diagnostic, dental, or surgical procedures or for adaptive support, as a medical protective device, or when voluntarily accepted by a patient	No	•Define applicable situations in restraint policy •Assess needs of individual patients •Monitor patients and attend to their needs during episode
Level 2: Carried out under medical staff approved protocols and executed by appropriately trained nurses	Yes	•Develop protocols for medical staff and nursing leadership approval •Train and designate staff competent to initiate protocols and apply, monitor, and terminate restraint use •Assess needs of individual patients •Monitor patients and attend to their needs during episodes •Measure, assess, and improve restraint use
Level 3: Carried out in response to time-limited orders from authorized, licensed independent practitioners in medical and surgical settings	Yes	•Develop policies on restrain application, including which licensed independent practitioners may issue orders •Assess needs of individual patients •Monitor patients and attend to their needs during episodes •Measure, assess, and improve restraint use
Level 4 (behavioral health care only): Carried out in response to time-limited orders by authorized, licensed independent practitioners (maximum length is four, two, or one hours, depending on patient's age, with extension of initial order possible for up to 24 hours)	Yes	•Develop policies on restraint application, including which licensed independent practitioners may issue order •Assess needs of individual patients •Monitor patients and attend to their needs during episodes •Measure, assess, and improve restraint use •Train and designate nurses competent to extend orders up to 24 hours

Consenting patients are legally required, however, to

- be a certain age (the age of consent in that state);
- have the intellectual capacity to provide knowing consent; and
- be aware of the purpose for restraint and the advantages and dangers associated with restraint (i.e., consent must be informed).

In the case of a patient who is determined to be legally incompetent and therefore cannot consent to restraint, the court will appoint a legal guardian who can consent on the patient's behalf. Subsequent restraint of that patient is then considered "voluntary," as if the patient had personally consented. Good clinical practice suggests that an effort be made to achieve the patient's understanding and consent anyway, even though it has no legal validity.

The issue of chemical restraint

Tranquilizing or sedative medications are sometimes used to control or eliminate undesirable behavior or movements and can produce some of the same negative effects as physical restraint. Therefore, some experts use the term *chemical restraint* to refer to such application of medications. HCFA, for example, defines chemical restraint in long-term care facilities as follows:

> *Chemical restraint: [Any] psychoactive drug administered for purposes of discipline or convenience, and not required to treat the resident's medical symptoms. (The Federal Register, 54: 5316–5336, 1989).*

Others apply the term *chemical restraint*—or at least apply the restrictions that go with the term—to any involuntary use of psychotropic or tranquilizing medication. Some authorities that recognize the term *chemical restraint* believe that restrictions similar to those applied to the use of physical restraint should apply to the use of chemical restraint as well. In fact, some states mandate special review of patients involuntarily treated with psychotropic medication.

But there are serious problems with defining chemical restraint specifically enough to clearly distinguish occasions in which restraint is intended from those in which restraint is not intended. For example, a tranquilizing drug might be administered to control a paranoid schizophrenic patient's outbursts of rage—one of the symptoms of paranoid schizophrenia. While this is, in a sense, chemical restraint, the basic purpose of the tranquilizing drug is to treat the underlying illness.

Even though regulations, standards, and restrictions similar to those for physical restraint might apply to chemical restraint in the future, the JCAHO and other leading authorities do not do so at present. For this reason, this book does not cover chemical restraint any further. Readers who are concerned with the JCAHO's regulation of psychotropic medication use should consult the standards that relate to medication use. (The JCAHO does not distinguish the use of psychotropics from the use of any other medications, although some states do.)

Defining seclusion

In contrast to defining restraint, it is relatively easy to define seclusion and to delineate which situations fall under its definition. In the updated 1999 *CAMH*, the JCAHO defines seclusion as follows:

> *Seclusion: The involuntary confinement of a person alone in a room where the person is physically prevented from leaving.*

Seclusion seldom is used in general healthcare settings. It is most often used in psychiatric hospitals and other behavioral healthcare settings in response to behavior that indicates patients might harm themselves or others. Seclusion is generally considered less restrictive and less severe than restraint since it allows patients a greater degree of movement.

Seclusion episodes are different from situations in which a patient willingly—or at least in agreement with the rules of the hospital—goes alone into a room that is left unlocked (what is often referred to as *time out*). Although a "time out" is sometimes used to deal with the same problems that seclusion deals with, it is considered far less restrictive than seclusion and usually does not have any special legal or clinical status. A situation in which a staff member is in a room with a patient does not technically meet the definition of seclusion either—even if the patient is prevented from leaving the room.

Combining restraint and seclusion under one set of standards

The JCAHO deals with restraint and seclusion as a single entity—applying the same standards to both procedures. Some states and hospitals treat the two procedures the same as well. For this reason, and because general hospitals and other healthcare organizations do not generally use seclusion, this book frequently uses the term *restraint* to cover both restraint and seclusion.

Treat all restraint episodes with care

Some restraint devices and approaches admittedly appear more intense and perhaps more dangerous than others. For example, a patient restrained with leather cuffs might suffer more skin damage—and possibly more psychological damage—than a patient restrained with cotton ties. And a patient restrained for a short period of time in an acute care setting while a medical procedure is performed is not likely to suffer to the same degree as a psychiatric patient restrained for days. But for all episodes of restraint, the potential for damage—especially psychological damage—still exists. So, although each episode is different, the level of care and attention should be the same for every episode.

Summary

- Each organization should develop its own definition of restraint, based on its own needs and unique situation. The definition must fall under the scope of the JCAHO's definition, but it will probably be far more specific.

- Good clinical practice and risk management suggest that most opt-outs should be treated with the same care and documentation efforts as restraint.

- Some opt-outs, however, are so brief and benign that they do not require any special attention if they are applied properly, such as when a patient is strapped to a stretcher during transportation.

- In addition to JCAHO standards, organizations must comply with state laws and regulations that apply to restraint.

Chapter Two

Common Uses of Restraint

Examining restraint in long-term care and acute care facilities

Why do healthcare professionals use restraint? There are many reasons—some questionable, others valid and even necessary. While restraint episodes can be harmful, they can also be lifesaving procedures.

In examining restraint use, we first have to distinguish between restraint use in long-term care facilities and restraint use in acute care facilities. Although staff in long-term care facilities routinely used restraint in the past, most knowledgeable professionals now agree that a properly designed and administered long-term care facility can greatly reduce and possibly even eliminate restraint use. Healthcare organizations can achieve the major objectives of restraint in long-term care—prevention of wandering and falls—with alternative methods that do not have the same potentially negative effects as restraint. For this reason, both the federal government and the JCAHO seriously restrict and discourage restraint use in long-term care settings.

Restraint use in acute care settings, however, is quite different from that in long-term care. Acute care settings fall easily into two groups: (1) medical and surgical treatment facilities, such as general hospitals and freestanding ambulatory surgery facilities; and (2) behavioral healthcare settings, such as psychiatric units in general hospitals, freestanding psychiatric hospitals, and mental health centers.

Many acute-care clinicians cannot conceive of treating patients without the availability of restraints (interestingly, though, some clinicians in medical and surgical facilities do not consider their use of restraint devices as falling within the category of restraint). Restraint is used in medical and surgical settings to prevent patients from accidentally or deliberately disturbing sutures, indwelling lines, and tubes. Restraint is also used less frequently to prevent a patient from getting out of a bed or chair and wandering or falling. Although, in theory, a facility can eliminate the need for restraint by significantly increasing staffing and limiting admissions to those patients who will almost certainly not need restraint, for obvious reasons, in these days of cost-cutting and regulation, such measures are seldom realistically available to a facility.

In behavioral healthcare settings, restraint is used to prevent patients from harming themselves or others, and sometimes to prevent disturbance or damage to the environment. Because some mentally ill or developmentally disabled persons can be unpredictable and irrational, behavioral healthcare facilities will rarely be able to establish restraint- or seclusion-free environments.

In contrast to long-term care settings, therefore, it appears that with only a few exceptions, acute-care organizations cannot hope to be completely restraint-free.

While this chapter discusses positive aspects of restraint use and the appropriateness of certain restraints, Chapter 3 explores negative aspects and problems associated with restraint use.

Preventing patients from harming themselves

The most obvious and common reason why staff apply restraint is to keep a patient from doing something that is directly or ultimately harmful to himself or herself. The training of countless healthcare professionals over the years has perpetuated this justification for restraint. However, only the following legitimate circumstances justify restraint to prevent patients from harming themselves.

Suicidal patients

State laws and regulations and hospital policies almost universally recognize using restraint to control acutely suicidal patients (states are the legal regulators of restraint use in the United States). Hospitals often admit acutely suicidal patients—either as a result of injuries from a suicide attempt or in an effort to avoid injury and treat the cause of the suicidal impulses. These suicidal patients—even those who are already seriously injured from a suicide attempt—might be so determined to kill themselves that the only relatively sure way of preventing further injury or death is through restraint. The suicidal impulse is often short-lived, however, and in that case the duration of restraint should be brief.

But the issue of whether or not to restrain suicidal patients is not black-and-white. When deciding whether to restrain such patients, healthcare professionals need to consider the negative psychological effects that restraint can have on suicidal patients who are already severely upset and depressed. Being tied up or locked in a room might seem like punishment, and might reduce a patient's self-esteem even further. Furthermore, placing suicidal patients in restraint might be dangerous, because experience has shown that intensely suicidal patients are sometimes able to escape from restraint and counter staff's preventive efforts—no matter how closely staff are watching. Restraint might even *stimulate* suicidal efforts. Finally, restraint use on suicidal patients also raises the philosophical and ethical question of whether a rational, determined individual has the right to commit suicide without interference and, if so, whether restraint use denies such right.

Injury without suicidal intent

Some patients who do not intend to commit suicide nonetheless engage in behaviors that might result in serious injury. Some mentally ill and developmentally disabled patients, for example, engage in repetitive activities such as banging their heads against a wall, scratching and tearing at their skin, or cutting themselves. These individuals might or might not be aware of what they are doing. Regardless, healthcare professionals believe that, in many cases, the only way to prevent such behavior is to use restraint. Such behaviors can be persistent and lead to weeks or even months of continuous restraint, however, which is a very dangerous and undesirable situation.

Diminished awareness or self-control

One legitimate use of restraint is for patients who have diminished awareness or self-control as a result of an illness or treatment—usually those receiving surgical or medical care. Such patients often interfere with treatment by engaging in harmful behaviors, including pulling out various tubes or lines inserted into parts of their bodies, removing bandages, pulling on sutures, or resisting the use of required medical equipment.

Fall prevention

Restraint can be used to help patients who are physically weak or suffering from diminished alertness in long-term care and behavioral healthcare facilities (elderly people compose the largest portion of this group). Such individuals can be prone to falling out of beds or chairs or falling while walking around—making them particularly susceptible to serious injury, such as hip fractures. Falls can occur, for example, when patients attempt to get out of bed at night to go to the bathroom or when patients are not strong enough to maintain a desired posture or position. Other falls occur when patients try to climb over bed rails to get out of bed. There are many effective alternatives to restraint for fall prevention, including bed alarms, low beds, improved night lighting, and non-skid floors (see Chapter 4 for more discussion of restraint alternatives).

Wandering prevention

Wanderers—patients who walk around the facility at inappropriate times or in inappropriate places or who leave their area or even the facility—might harm themselves or others. For example, wanderers might get lost and expose themselves to hunger, thirst, physical injury, or other hazards. They might also invade the privacy of, upset, or even attack other patients. Restraint is one means to prevent wandering. Many experts question the appropriateness of using restraint to prevent wandering, however, because there are many other, less-restrictive means to control it (see Chapter 4).

Preventing patients from harming others

Some patients—usually those who are mentally ill or developmentally disabled—are compelled to physically attack others. Attacks might be triggered when, for example, the person who attacks

- experiences a perceptual mistake about the identity of the victim;
- misunderstands the meaning of another person's action;
- loses control of himself or herself, such as in a temper tantrum;

- is intoxicated or delirious; or
- exhibits automatic and unconscious behavior, such as a seizure.

Restraint provides a relatively safe way to achieve control over such patients in many healthcare settings—particularly behavioral healthcare settings and emergency rooms. An effective nursing staff can quickly place such a patient in restraint, reducing the risk of injury to the patient and others. Without the availability of restraint, it is difficult to conceive of a safe way of dealing with hostile, combative patients who are resistant to all psychological efforts. (Of course, seclusion and tranquilizing medications are alternatives, but these are usually considered either a form of restraint or so closely related to restraint that there is no meaningful difference. Furthermore, medication use has a number of drawbacks: it does not work instantly, it can produce serious side effects or even death, and the patient's physical condition or other medications might preclude the use of the necessary medication.)

"Therapeutic" holding

Therapeutic holding is a potentially dangerous restraint technique in which one or more staff members hold a patient's limbs so the patient cannot strike out. In the heading above, we have placed the term in quotation marks to signal that therapeutic holding is often not "therapeutic" at all, but is more like wrestling than holding. Staff-to-patient physical contact frequently occurs when staff attempt to place an uncooperative patient in restraint. In most instances, holding is brief and is a step toward definitive treatment. However, experience has shown that many of the injuries and deaths associated with restraint occur during therapeutic holding because there is a high risk that the holding maneuver will turn into a physical struggle between the staff members and the patient.

Staff might also effectively use therapeutic holding in place of restraint for children—usually in a temper tantrum—without risking significant danger to either the child or staff. The child might be lifted off the ground and/or placed in a bear hug. The hold should be brief when it is used to control a temper tantrum.

Therapeutic holding is also used as an alternative to mechanical restraint. In this situation, a number of staff members—often five or six—gather around the patient and get control over his or her limbs and trunk. They then physically maintain the hold until the patient no longer needs restraint, which might last an hour or more. The rationale behind this use of holding is to communicate to the patient the staff's concern for the patient and interest in staying with the patient through the crisis. Many feel that using holding in this way is less cold and distancing than mechanical restraint.

However, we strongly advise against using therapeutic holding as an alternative to mechanical restraint for several reasons:

- The patient might actively resist holding for a prolonged period of time, placing him or her at risk of exhaustion, overheating, and dehydration.
- Prolonged holding increases the probability of significant physical injury to the patient or staff.
- Prolonged holding increases the possibility of psychological damage to both the patient and staff, who might view each other as antagonists during the struggle.
- A physical struggle between a large patient and a small number of staff might cause one or more staff members to injure the patient in an attempt to keep the patient from overpowering the staff.

Because it is such a dangerous procedure, therapeutic holding requires special scrutiny before it is incorporated into organization policy and carried out on patients. It also deserves close consideration because it is not defined by the JCAHO (and is therefore excluded from coverage under the JCAHO standards). To try to prevent an escalation of conflict during therapeutic holding, sufficient staff should be present when preparing to get a patient under control so that the patient can clearly see that physical struggle will not prevent restraint. Sufficient staffing also prevents the need for hand-to-hand grappling between patients and staff.

The JCAHO does not require a physician's order for therapeutic holding, because at present, it does not consider therapeutic holding to be restraint. Consequently, there is no documentation requirement. Nonetheless, for good clinical care, organizations using holding should have a policy that requires a physician's order and careful documentation. An effective safety measure during holding is to require a staff member (such as the team leader) to act as an observer. This person can complete the documentation as a physically uninvolved staff member and might also provide assistance if the situation threatens to spin out of control.

Takedown as a control measure

When staff need to restrain resistant patients, they must sometimes force patients to comply. In such cases, staff often place a patient on the floor to achieve control over the patient's limbs—a procedure called takedown. In most organizations, the decision to use takedown is up to the nursing staff and does not require a separate physician's order. Staff participating in a takedown risk their own well-being in a confrontation that might call for all-out force. Therefore, takedown should be carried out in conjunction with de-escalation to the greatest possible extent (see p. 50 for more information on de-escalation).

Takedown is probably one of the most dangerous aspects of restraint for patients and staff. Therefore, most hospitals provide special training for some or all of their nursing staff in takedown methods. But, as with therapeutic holding, training should include appropriate psychological preparation; too often, training emphasizes effective physical execution without instruction on the appropriate attitude. Staff must see takedown as clinical care, not as rule enforcement.

Walking restraint

Some severely ill psychiatric or developmentally disabled patients strike at those around them without apparent reason or warning. Such behavior can persist for weeks or months. One alternative approach to four-point restraint for these patients—clearly an undesirable and dangerous approach—is to restrain the patient's arms, but not legs, called *walking restraint*. This permits the patient to freely walk around the treatment setting and participate at least to a limited extent.

Walking restraint can reduce some of the long-term risks associated with keeping a patient restrained in a bed or chair, such as loss of strength, circulatory problems, and complete dependence on others (see Chapter 3 for a discussion of negative aspects of restraint). But restraining a patient's arms makes him or her defenseless against attacks by other patients, and might be considered a violation of the patient's privacy. Furthermore, this type of restraint might tempt staff to prolong its use because it is less restrictive and harmful than full restraint, even though it is actually more difficult for staff to keep track of and monitor the needs of these patients as they walk around.

De-escalation as a means of restraint

Although it is not technically a means of restraint, de-escalation is so important and intertwined with restraint that it deserves some discussion here. De-escalation is a method of resolving a confrontational, violence-prone situation without the use of physical force or control. It is an acquired, teachable skill that uses verbal and nonverbal communication to calm people. De-escalation is typically used in behavioral healthcare settings and hospital emergency rooms for violent or out-of-control patients. A related technique, called *distraction*, is useful to staff in general acute care settings in response to a confused or physically distressed patient, rather than an angry or fearful one.

Preventing damage to property or the milieu

Some states and the JCAHO permit hospitals to restrain patients to prevent damage to furniture, parts of the building, and even to the social tranquility of the setting. State laws and regulations vary, however, and the JCAHO requires that organizations clinically justify such restraint. If staff use restraint to protect the environment, hospital policy and entries in patient records must provide clear clinical justification.

The threat of damage to property is easy to identify and act upon. Behavior that disrupts social tranquility—such as disruptive noisemaking, use of vulgar or threatening language, or refusal to obey rules—usually requires more subjective evaluation, but it is considered appropriate cause for restraint in some settings. Organizations should take great care to document evidence that restraint is justified in these situations, however, and is not used simply to punish for expressing unpopular views or using unpleasant language, which is undesirable but not dangerous.

Contingent restraint

Healthcare organizations sometimes use restraint as part of a *behavior management program* (also referred to as *behavior modification* or *behavior therapy*). We define such a program thus: a treatment program usually developed by a doctorate-level qualified professional that applies the principles of learning theory, including positive and negative reinforcement, to reduce or eliminate undesirable behavior. These programs are usually used in long-term behavioral healthcare facilities and are used to treat particularly difficult patients.

In a behavior management program, a patient might be automatically restrained (without an order) as a negative reinforcement for a particular behavior—a practice called *contingent restraint*. Patient behaviors that warrant behavior management programs are typically extremely resistant to change and are seriously deleterious, such as

- head-banging and other self-destructive behaviors;
- frequent, unpredictable, and dangerous attacks on other patients or staff; and
- unpredictable and repeated ingestion of dangerous substances.

Behavior management programs that use negative reinforcement or aversive stimuli are rare and closely regulated by state law or other regulations.

A behavior management program that is professionally acceptable is based on a detailed behavior analysis and a plan that is prepared by an appropriately trained professional. If restraint or seclusion is used as part of a behavioral management program, staff should apply it in strict accord with the plan or protocol. Restraint used as outlined in the plan does not require a doctor's order.

Chapter Three

Problems, Risks, and Disadvantages of Restraint Use

To restrain or not to restrain?

As Chapter 2 discusses, common clinical practice supports the use of restraint in a wide variety of situations. Some legal experts also support frequent restraint use to avoid negligence claims that often result when unrestrained patients are accidentally injured by falls or similar incidents (see p. 64 for more discussion of this type of liability).

On the other hand, there is an increasing consensus among experts that restraint does more damage to patients and staff than is prevented by its use. Some go as far as to suggest that it might be best for hospitals to eliminate restraint use entirely. The media, the JCAHO, and several healthcare associations have amassed ample evidence of the injuries and harm restraint causes, ranging from mild physical or psychological injury to death. Although the frequency of restraint-related injuries is difficult to determine, such injuries are definitely not a rare occurrence: A significant number of patients die every year while in restraints; many of these die *because of* being restrained.

A middle course between the two positions is probably best for hospitals and other clinical organizations. An organization should use restraint when it is clearly needed and there is no realistic alternative, but it should treat restraint as a highly dangerous procedure, use numerous safeguards when applying it, and maintain excellent records.

Organizations should also use all possible preventive and safety measures when applying restraint-like procedures, or opt-outs (see Chapter 1, p. 37 for more information on opt-outs). Even in the face of anti-restraint statistics and evidence—and even though some studies indicate a reduction in serious injuries after facilities become restraint-free—some organizations still use restraint with little regard to the potential detrimental consequences.

This chapter discusses the drawbacks, risks, and disadvantages that are associated with restraint and seclusion, which every organization that is considering or using restraint or seclusion should examine. Many of the problems do not have easy solutions, and even experts disagree on the subject. This discussion is based on observation of restraint and seclusion in numerous hospitals and on discussions with many professionals. In this chapter, restraint refers to any situation in which restraint-like procedures or seclusion are used. That is, in addition to restraint and seclusion, it covers those procedures, opt-outs, that the JCAHO excludes from the restraint standards.

Physical injury or death

The most serious negative effects of restraint are physical injury and death, for both patients *and staff*. The following section discusses several reasons why patients might suffer physical injury or death from restraint.

Patient actions

A patient might suffer injury or death while simply trying to change position or by struggling against a restraint—often in an attempt to get free. Although complete statistics are not available, there are numerous documented cases of patients strangling on vests, falling out of bed after climbing over bed rails, or injuring themselves while squirming to get out of ties. There are several recent reports that restrained patients burned to death after attempting to burn their restraints off or light a cigarette. In one case, the restrained patient's roommate also was killed. Patients or staff are also sometimes injured when staff must use force to place a patient in a restraint against his or her will.

Patient actions can result in dehydration. Patients who struggle while restrained or by resisting the application of restraint, for example, can become severely dehydrated from perspiring and overheating. It is also not uncommon for restrained patients to refuse liquids. Therefore, if staff are misled by a patient's denial of thirst and do not give sufficient fluids, the patient will likely become dehydrated.

Dehydration can cause severe physical problems, such as hypotension, weakness, cardiovascular collapse, or even death—particularly in patients who are elderly and/or are already ill.

Improper application of restraint

The improper application of restraint can cause injury or death. For example,

- a patient might partially slip out of and strangle on an improperly applied vest;
- a restraint that is fastened to the improper point on a bed or chair might tighten and injure a patient when the bed is elevated or the chair is moved;
- a restraint that is applied too loosely might allow a patient to partially escape, leaving the patient in a dangerous and vulnerable position; or
- a restraint applied too tightly might abrade skin, cut off circulation, or damage joints.

Limited movement and consequent dependence

Physical restraints that limit a patient's freedom of movement and ability to care for himself or herself can cause physical injuries, such as those described below. Most such injuries usually occur only after a prolonged period of restraint, but skin damage can occur in as little as a few minutes if the patient struggles or if staff improperly apply restraints.

- ***Dehydration:*** Patients in restraint who must rely on others to provide liquids for them are especially susceptible to dehydration and its potential consequences, as outlined above.
- ***Choking:*** Patients in restraint—especially those who must remain on their backs—are at risk of choking on vomit, food, liquid, or even saliva. Patients who were restrained face down have also asphyxiated when they could not raise their heads enough to have a clear airway.

- ***Loss of strength and mobility:*** Patients might also lose physical strength, muscle mass, and agility, or develop contracture of joints as a result of restrictions that prolonged restraint places on their movement. If staff do not quickly treat and reverse such conditions through increased exercise and movement, the conditions can become disabling. Even with exercise and movement, however, successful treatment is difficult in many cases because the general condition of patients is too poor.

- ***Incontinence:*** Restrained patients might experience a loss of bowel or bladder control if they are not given access to the toilet frequently enough. Although this loss of control is temporary in most cases, lasting only as long as the patient does not have adequate toilet access, it can sometimes become permanent in patients whose control is already weak. And elderly patients are often predisposed to incontinence because of a urinary tract or cognitive problem. In any case, an episode of incontinence can have serious psychological effects.

Injury from other patients

In some psychiatric facilities, patients in restraint are vulnerable to attack by other patients, such as when a patient is in a walking restraint or is restrained in a bed that is accessible to other patients. Ideally, such attacks should not occur because staff are constantly observing and have control over the situation. Regardless, prudence and the fact that allowing other patients to observe a person in restraint can be considered a violation of that person's privacy suggest that restrained patients should never be accessible to other patients.

Psychological injury

In addition to physical injury, restraint can cause psychological harm. Although psychological injury is a potential danger especially to behavioral health patients (many of whom are particularly vulnerable because restraint is a relatively frequent and prolonged event), medical or surgical patients are also at risk.

Probably the foremost adverse psychological effects of restraint or seclusion for adults are a sharp decrease in self-esteem and a negative self-image. Adults are accustomed to a significant degree of independence and the ability to determine the flow of events in their lives. Restraint interferes with even the most routine decisions, such as what to wear and when to eat, and subjects patients to complete dependence on someone else to meet their most basic needs.

A restrained patient is in danger of coming to see himself or herself as dependent, childlike, and under the control of others. As a result, restrained patients often become demoralized and depressed very quickly, which is especially damaging for restrained patients who, in most cases, already have a tenuous self-concept. In addition, a patient's willingness or ability to carry out adult tasks can be so greatly impaired that he or she might not be willing or able to resume an adult role when released from restraint.

Restraint is particularly difficult for some medical and surgical patients who must depend on others for their basic needs and have little control over many aspects of their lives because of their illness. Medical and surgical patients who have been restrained report that the experience led to feelings of terror, helplessness, and extreme psychological discomfort.

Even patients whose awareness of their surroundings is marginal because of cognitive deterioration, such as confused or delirious patients, might experience a fear of helplessness and abandonment from restraint. Restraint might even cause such patients to become disoriented or psychotic because it diminishes their contact with their surroundings (some patients even believe that they are in prison or are being punished), which further increases their distress and confusion.

Although there are many effective measures that can help reduce the risk of physical injury to patients in restraint, there are few preventive measures for psychological harm. The longer a patient is restrained, the greater the likelihood of psychological injury.

Social damage

In addition to physical and psychological harm, restraint can also have negative social effects. Patients who are restrained for a short period of time because of medical or surgical procedures are likely to suffer little if any social stigma, but behavioral patients who experience long or frequent episodes of restraint—or even single episodes of seclusion—can suffer significant negative social effects. A patient might, for example,

- experience feelings of isolation from other patients after he or she is released from restraint;
- become depressed or feel disgraced—causing him or her to withdraw from social interaction;
- become so dependent that he or she cannot interact as an adult;
- become clinically disoriented as a result of losing track of the date, day of the week, time, important current events, and other similar items while in restraint; and
- have difficulty rejoining his or her group of peers.

In addition, even patients who are not restrained, but who see other patients in restraint or seclusion, might not understand the need for restraint or seclusion and might fear that something similar will happen to them.

Differences between the negative effects of physical restraint and those of seclusion

Seclusion is usually considered to be less restrictive and less stressful to patients than restraint. Seclusion is generally closer to everyday life than restraint. Even though the patient is locked up in a room, the patient can still move around and is able to control many details of personal preference, such as adjusting clothing, scratching an itch, etc. Seclusion also presents no danger to skin integrity, joint movement, or muscle condition.

But many of the negative effects and dangers associated with physical restraint occur with seclusion as well. For example, secluded patients are at risk of dehydration and overheating from severe physical exertion, such as by attempting to force open a door or window. In addition, secluded patients are actually often at greater risk of self-injury than patients in physical restraint.

Many seclusion rooms, for example, have solid, unpadded, and roughly surfaced walls that patients can rub their skin or hurl themselves against—actions that can seriously injure or even kill patients if they are done powerfully enough. Secluded patients who are not under constant observation can also hang themselves by using clothing as a noose. And some seclusion rooms have appliances or devices built into them, such as radiators, sprinkler heads, lights, and window grills, that patients also can use to injure themselves. For example, a determined patient can easily tie a noose to a radiator knob or doorknob and hang himself or herself by sitting down forcefully.

Patients in seclusion are likely to be more isolated than patients in physical restraint because they are usually alone in a room. And secluded patients are usually observed remotely, while patients in physical restraint are usually in frequent or constant contact with observers. It is easier for overworked staff to decrease the frequency with which they observe secluded patients than physically restrained patients, since secluded patients are not as helpless and are basically locked away out of sight and hearing.

Other issues and problems associated with restraint and seclusion

In addition to the potential for physical, psychological, and social injury to patients and staff, restraint and seclusion present other issues and problems that hospitals should address.

Unnecessary, inappropriate, and improper restraint and seclusion

One of the main issues and problems associate with restraint is that staff often use restraint and seclusion for the wrong reasons or do not apply it properly, such as in the following situations.

Restraint used as punishment

Few healthcare professionals approve of or defend the restraint used as punishment. Yet in practice it is sometimes difficult to distinguish between restraint used as a preventive measure and restraint used as punishment. This issue arises most frequently in psychiatric settings, but it can occur in general hospital and other healthcare settings as well.

When a psychiatric patient attacks a staff member, for example, the patient is usually immediately restrained. There might be little or no consideration of whether the patient's anger—or whatever situation provoked the attack—has run its course (in which case there would be no continued danger of attack). Although the patient's record in such a case would likely indicate that restraint was used to protect others, the real reason for using restraint might really have been to teach the patient a lesson—staff might feel that the physical and mental discomfort of restraint will discourage the patient from repeating the undesirable behavior—or to offer staff a means of revenge.

But staff should use restraint only to prevent behavior or actions that they fear a patient will carry out, not because of what a patient has done. Restraint should not be used as punishment except when it is used as contingent restraint, which requires a formal behavior control plan designed by an appropriately qualified professional (see Chapter 2, p. 51 for more information on contingent restraint).

Threat of restraint as a means of control

Patients who are at least somewhat rational and able to control themselves will usually try to control their behavior to avoid restraint. For this reason, staff in psychiatric facilities and other healthcare settings might sometimes threaten to use restraint to reduce undesirable behavior. Of course, such threats are effective only if patients know that these threats are occasionally carried out. Therefore, like restraint used as punishment, threats of restraint are not acceptable.

Using restraint in response to short staffing

All types of organizations sometimes lack sufficient staff to monitor the activities of every patient at all times. But without monitoring, patients can engage in such deleterious behavior as removing tubes, lines, and bandages; wandering around treatment units; falling; attacking other patients; or even attempting suicide. When any of these behaviors occurs, a hospital and its staff can be held accountable.

Staff might use restraint to reduce the risk of such deleterious patient behavior in response to a staffing shortage. Or even worse, staff might be tempted to use restraint during a staffing shortage to keep patients from requesting care or taking actions that add to the staff workload. While this use of restraint might successfully decrease the short-term risk and workload for the hospital and staff, it increases the risk of long-term damage to patients.

Relying on restraint might inhibit the identification of root causes

Patient behaviors that restraint is intended to control almost always have multiple causes and multiple solutions. Using restraint as a preventive measure or as an inappropriate response to patient behavior might hinder the recognition of environmental problems that could be resolved in a more positive way.

Analysis of restraint use must always include consideration of "root causes"—the factors that led to an episode of restraint—and the availability of alternatives. Searching for the root cause of a restraint episode is not only good clinical practice that can help to reduce restraint use but also can benefit patient care in general by identifying fundamental causes of distress.

For example, using restraint in an attempt to control a patient's agitation in a psychiatric hospital might mask a real, preventable problem, such as inadequate medication or poor communication among patients in group meetings. Or, in a general hospital, frequent restraint use in a medical unit on patients who have nasogastric tubes might hide excessive use of such tubes or failure to remove the tubes when they are no longer needed. Conducting a root-cause analysis could help reduce restraint use by unmasking and correcting such detrimental environmental factors.

Legal issues to consider

In addition to considering the potentially harmful effects of restraint and the importance of avoiding its use for inappropriate reasons, hospitals must pay attention to a number of legal issues as well. Legal requirements regarding the application of restraint are complex and demanding and vary from state to state. In many cases, state requirements are stricter than the JCAHO standards, so organizational leaders should consult with an attorney who is an expert in their state's healthcare law when developing an organizational policy on restraint and seclusion.

The levels at which healthcare practice and the legal system interact on the issue of restraint can be grouped into four main categories:

- patient consent;
- the legal authority to "imprison" a person outside the criminal justice system;
- organizational liability for using restraint inappropriately; and
- organizational liability for failing to use restraint.

Patient consent

Unless warned, patients almost never expect restraint to be part of their course of treatment. But when it is apparent that a patient might need to be restrained or secluded, it is best to explain the need for restraint to the patient (or legal guardian, as explained below) and to obtain consent to apply restraint or seclusion well before the need arises. If a patient is both clinically and legally competent to provide informed consent to restraint or seclusion and does so, clinical staff are free to use these procedures when they are indicated. If a patient has been declared legally incompetent and has an appointed legal guardian who is legally authorized to make decisions as if the patient were making them personally, then the guardian can provide consent.

In the majority of situations in which restraint is necessary, however, patients are unable to consent because, at the time, they cannot understand or process the information about the procedure, or cannot clearly indicate consent. Often, restraint or seclusion is necessary to protect life or limb. In these situations, staff must apply restraint without specific consent, and at best with the implied consent based upon the patient's acceptance of the overall treatment. If a patient has provided a general consent to treatment, this should not be considered a specific consent to restraint. (A specific consent to restraint excludes the episode from coverage under the JCAHO restraint standards.)

If the patient's family members are present, it is a good idea to alert them to the situation and enlist their support, even though they cannot consent on behalf of the patient unless given legal authority to do so. Keep in mind, however, that this can be a confusing medico-legal situation: strictly speaking, information about a patient's condition cannot be shared with relatives without the patient's consent.

Advance directives

With medical and surgical patients, *advance directives* refers to the decision a patient can make upon admission to a hospital regarding the extent of resuscitation and life support he or she desires in the event of a life-threatening situation. This is not related in any way to restraint. But with psychiatric patients—particularly those who are severely and chronically ill—the term refers to the opportunity to decide during a rational period what the course of treatment should be during a subsequent irrational period. During the rational period, a psychiatric patient can be asked to consent to future treatment measures and can knowingly weigh the pros and cons of restraint or seclusion. For example, using advance directives can give a patient the option of choosing to be heavily medicated, or restrained, or secluded. Depending on the patient's legal status, the patient's consent may well be legally valid several weeks or months later, when the patient needs restraint or seclusion and is beyond the ability to give informed consent.

There are several advantages to the use of advance directives. Involving the patient in determining the course of treatment is required for most diseases and is always good clinical practice, when feasible, for psychiatric patients. And JCAHO standards do not apply to episodes of restraint or seclusion for which legally valid consent is obtained, which can simplify paperwork. Finally, advance directives can minimize the demeaning effects of restraint or seclusion, since the patient is involved in the choice to use these approaches rather than having them imposed.

Use of force and imprisonment without judicial recourse

Restraint can be an injury-preventing or even lifesaving procedure, and it almost always protects patients or staff from serious harm. But consider this: A healthcare organization is probably the only place in America where an ordinary, free individual can be suddenly, involuntarily, and legally imprisoned, tied down, or subjected to painful procedures and have almost no immediate recourse or appeal.

Even an individual arrested on criminal charges has the right to a lawyer, quick legal review by a judge or magistrate, and an opportunity to make a case for immediate release until trial. But patients have none of these immediate protections because state laws permit medical personnel acting in an emergency to take extreme action without the patient's consent and without legal review until many days or even months later. Out of respect for the expertise and dedication of its workers, the healthcare system has been granted enormous power over those to whom it provides assistance. Professionals in the healthcare system have always done their best to deserve this respect and power, but they must never forget the special authority that society gives to them and should constantly examine their actions to ensure that they do not betray society's trust.

Liability for inappropriate use of restraint

The inappropriate use of restraint can be the basis for a patient lawsuit against a healthcare organization, although such a scenario is rare. Even so, organizations must factor this situation into the development of their policies and staff training. The bases for a lawsuit, which could include criminal charges, includes assault, battery, false imprisonment, and carrying out treatment without consent. In addition, if a patient was injured during an episode of restraint or seclusion, the organization can be held liable for that injury, even if restraint use was clinically justified. The best way to avoid a lawsuit is to document the need for restraint or seclusion and apply it in accordance with state laws and regulations.

Liability for failure to use restraint

Many healthcare professionals believe that they can be held liable if they fail to restrain a patient who is in danger of falling, wandering, or self-injury. This belief applies especially to situations in which the patient is at risk of suicide, even though this means applying a psychologically stressful procedure to a patient who is already in a state of extreme agitation, stress, and low self-esteem. Lawsuits have been filed in cases in which nonapplication of restraint was followed by injury. However, statistical studies show that such lawsuits are rare, and many experts believe that restraint causes more injuries than nonapplication of restraint. Generally, the risk of liability might be greater when restraint is applied than in situations in which restraint is not applied.

Chapter Four

Improving Practice

Monitoring and improving restraint use should be a key activity

Because restraint and seclusion are dangerous, high-risk procedures, healthcare organizations should carefully evaluate how they use them. Questions that can help in this process include:

- Are we using restraint too frequently?
- Are we providing enough alternatives to restraint?
- Are our staffing levels appropriate? and
- Are we training staff well enough?

To answer such questions, organizations must gather data, assess it, and compare it to other organizations and to their own prior patterns of restraint use. Only then can organizations identify problems and make improvements. This chapter discusses the appropriate frequency of restraint use, presents ideas on how to evaluate its application, and describes ways in which organizations can reduce restraint use.

Determining the frequency of restraint use is difficult

How often is restraint or seclusion used in any given facility? This is not an easy question to answer, since the frequency of use is usually calculated from reports in medical records, which do not necessarily accurately or completely report what actually happened with patients. One critically important study that was based on actual observation of patients—not just on patient records—found that over one-third of restraint episodes were not documented. The obvious implication is that the frequency of restraint use that most studies report is probably underestimated.

In addition, since there are many ways to calculate the frequency of restraint use, published reports are often not comparable. For example, while some studies count the proportion of admitted patients who ever experience restraint during a hospital stay, others calculate the number of restraint episodes per number of patient days. Furthermore, the definition of a restraint episode varies among organizations. For example, some organizations count when a patient is continuously restrained through the course of several order renewals as one episode because it is continuous, while others count each renewal of the order as a separate episode. Similarly, if a patient is released from restraint but then placed back in restraint without a new order, some organizations count this as one episode of restraint, while others count it as two.

Because of this lack of comparability, many experts discuss a range of frequencies rather than a particular frequency. Published comments on the frequency of restraint use in nursing homes, acute care general hospitals, and psychiatric hospitals report ranges from 0% to 66% of all admitted patients. (Overall, the consensus is in the 20% area for general and psychiatric hospitals.) Although frequency comparisons with national groups or with similar hospitals are useful, the best comparisons are internal comparisons, such as a before-and-after comparison when a new restraint prevention program is initiated.

How to monitor your own use of restraint

An organization should formally evaluate its restraint use to get a better idea of whether its restraint episodes are clinically justified. The JCAHO requires organizations to perform regular statistical monitoring of the frequency of restraint use and of the characteristics of individual restraint episodes.

There are two approaches to evaluating restraint use: the case-by-case review and statistical quality control. Both case-by-case review and statistical quality control can be useful, particularly when used together.

Case-by-case review

In a case-by-case review—also called in some facilities *review of critical incidents,* or *peer review*—one or more clinical experts examine the details of restraint episodes to determine if patient care was adequate and appropriate. While this approach may be used to evaluate every restraint episode or a random sample of episodes, it usually involves reviewing only those cases that had an adverse outcome.

However, although the JCAHO did, at one time, permit organizations to limit quality improvement efforts only to those cases that had quality problems (i.e., adverse events), it now requires organizations to perform regular statistical measurement of quality—regardless of whether adverse events occur. In other words, the JCAHO maintains that the absence of a disaster does not mean that the status quo is necessarily good enough. A hospital should constantly assess its quality of care and consider improvements even if no major problems occur. Furthermore, even if initial baseline quality level measures are acceptable, regular monitoring and data assessment should continue. (This JCAHO requirement applies not only to restraint but to performance improvement in general.)

This review of adverse events involves a careful analysis of all available information about the problematic restraint episode—what the JCAHO refers to as intensive assessment—to determine what went wrong and why. Review of adverse events might go beyond examination of documentation and include interviews with involved staff or even with patients.

Case-by-case review is almost always subjective because experts evaluate care by asking themselves: "Is this good care?" or "Would I have treated this case in the same way?" If the answer is yes, the expert designates the care as satisfactory; if the answer is no, the expert labels the care as inadequate, and the clinician who applied restraint is typically asked to defend the quality of care. On the other hand, case-by-case evaluation can be made at least partially objective when experts apply a predetermined set of standards to screen cases and then scrutinize only those cases that do not meet the predetermined standards.

The corrective action stemming from a review of such cases often focuses on individual practitioners who are held responsible for poor care, and that action is often punitive in nature. Some organizations, however, use the case-by-case approach in a new, more systematic way that involves examining the complete sequence of events that led up to a restraint episode. This method is essentially the root-cause analysis process that the JCAHO requires for sentinel events. This approach is useful because it emphasizes inherent system flaws rather than individual errors.

Statistical quality control: Gather and analyze data

Another approach to evaluating restraint use is statistical quality control, which involves collecting information about every restraint episode and analyzing it statistically. This approach can produce an objective, quantitative cross-section of an organization's practices that is comparable to other organizations' practices or to the organization's own practices over time. The resulting corrective action from statistical quality control usually focuses on changing the care provision system rather than reprimanding individual practitioners.

Although detailed information about how to examine restraint statistics is beyond the scope of this book, the following guidelines should help readers understand the basics. Every organization should also have at least one staff member who is familiar with statistical analysis techniques.

The best way to carry out statistical analysis is to evaluate the rate of restraint use in relation to certain variables. For example, some of the variables that an organization might examine in relation to the frequency of restraint include

- characteristics of patients who undergo restraint, such as age, sex, diagnosis, predominant symptoms, and length of hospital stay;

- characteristics of staff member(s) who were most involved in initiating restraint, such as their age, sex, professional background, professional experience, and past rate of involvement in restraint (in most instances, a physician orders restraint, but in reality, his or her order might be a ratification of a decision someone else made);

- characteristics of the restraint episode, such as the time of day, precipitating incident, method of restraint, and length of time in restraint;
- the quality and completeness of the documentation;
- preventive strategies that were attempted—including medication—that failed to prevent the need for restraint; and
- the outcome of the restraint, such as any injury to the patient or staff, continued need for restraint, or an improvement in condition following restraint.

In addition to the above, an organization might identify other variables that are useful to consider. The review of data relating to these variables should provide valuable information for improving restraint use—including determining possible alternatives. An organization should decide which variables it will examine before collecting data, because experience has shown that data collection that relies on routine medical records content often suffers if personnel do not know in advance exactly which items they should record. Some records will be found to be missing the needed items.

Because medical records might not accurately report what happened during restraint episodes, it is worth considering conducting a study to compare the frequency and characteristics of restraint use calculated from direct observation of patients to the frequency and characteristics calculated from the same patients' medical records.

Statistical comparisons

An organization should compare its statistical data on restraint use against other sets of similar data—from either internal or external sources. Such comparisons help to uncover problematic areas. For example, by tracking and comparing its own restraint use monthly, an organization might find that its frequency of restraint use per 1,000 patient days is significantly higher in one month than previous months. Or an organization might compare its restraint data to a similar organization's through a database that the organization subscribes to. The organization might also elect to exchange data directly with one or more agreeable associations or to compare its data to published information. An organization might find, for example, that its average length of restraint is significantly longer than the average at other facilities.

An organization should be aware that when it compares rates of restraint use, it might sometimes have to adjust the rates to account for factors that change over time and seem likely to affect the interpretation of the rates. For example, if the average age of patients in a psychiatric unit is 35, but for some reason a large number of patients under age 20 are admitted to the unit in the course of a particular month, the age difference could impact the frequency of restraint use. Similarly, if one hospital has a consistently higher rate of restraint than another does, those interpreting the data should consider differences in patient populations in the two facilities and make appropriate statistical adjustments.

In addition, measurements should always be interpreted carefully. Statisticians know that even when two separate measurements of the same item are compared (such as two measurements of the length of the same table), there is always a discrepancy in the results. Such a phenomenon is referred to as *random variation* because the variations or differences between measurements occur in a random manner. Random variations can be disregarded because they do not represent real differences.

On the other hand, an organization cannot disregard variations that stem from real differences in practice, patient characteristics, or other essential items. To distinguish random variation from real differences, an organization should use well-known, simple statistical formulas that determine with a high degree of probability what type of difference exists between any two sets of data.

Take action

When an organization's case-by-case review and statistical analysis of restraint reveals a problem, the organization must take action. Typically, an organization appoints a group—or task force—to investigate the problem, determine if further action is necessary, and, if so, recommend a solution. The individuals who compose a task force usually have a variety of backgrounds, but many of them have assignments in areas in which the problem occurs. For example, to investigate a restraint problem, nursing personnel at several different skill levels who work in units where restraint is used should make up a large part of the task force.

Root-cause analysis

A common method task forces use to investigate restraint episodes is to conduct a root-cause analysis. A root-cause analysis begins with the assumption—what many would consider a fact—that any problem has multiple causes. While some causes are tangential to the overall problem and do not require investigation, others—the root causes—are significant contributors to the problem. If the root causes are resolved, the problem can be wholly, or at least partially, solved. The first step, then, is to list and show the relationships among all the possible factors the group can think of (note this focuses on *factors*, not *people*).

For example, a root-cause analysis of excessive injuries restrained patients sustained on a particular medical unit might identify the root causes of the injuries as (1) the severe illness of the patients; (2) the design of the unit, which prevents observation of restrained patients from the nurses' station; (3) use of restraint materials that are abrasive to the skin; and (4) the use of nurses who are from an agency and are not regular staff members. Based on the analysis, the task force can make appropriate recommendations to the administrative body, which has the authority to make the changes. In this case, some of the root causes can be easily and inexpensively eliminated, such as replacing abrasive restraint materials, but other causes are difficult or impossible to change, such as the design of the medical unit.

Reducing the frequency of restraint use

As other chapters have discussed, because of the risks and negative effects associated with restraint, clinical prudence and expert consensus dictate that healthcare practitioners avoid the use of restraint when possible. The JCAHO now requires organizations to take measures to reduce restraint use and to justify—very clearly—why restraint was necessary when used.

There is, in fact, a trend in healthcare toward decreasing the use of restraint. Many studies indicate a great capacity for organizations to reduce restraint use, and campaigns to reduce restraint use in facilities have even resulted in restraint-free environments. Hospitals that make an effort to use alternatives to restraint usually succeed. And many long-term care facilities have demonstrated that, even though it seemed they were using restraint appropriately and minimally, determined efforts to reduce restraint use produced a lower frequency or complete cessation of it.

Exactly which alternatives to restraint an organization should use depends upon the nature of the facility, its patient population, and staff characteristics and training. Each facility has to examine for itself what it should try to achieve in restraint reduction and what might be the best route to achieve that goal. Some of the methods that have worked to reduce restraint are provided in Figure 4.1. Several alternatives are also discussed below.

Have appropriate staffing and staff training

Restraint is often the obvious method to prevent or stop certain undesirable behaviors, such as wandering. Wandering occurs more easily when staff are not around to observe and interact with patients, so busy staff—especially those whose units are short-staffed—are tempted to tie patients into bed so the patients cannot wander.

But in the long run, this use of restraint is actually false economy. Restrained patients require *more* intensive observation and staff time than ordinary patients do. Failure to carry out appropriate observation of restrained patients inevitably leads to serious injury to patients, and possible sanctions by an accrediting or inspection agency.

Facilities should make sure that they not only have an adequate number of staff members, but also that the staff members are well trained, since staff need to be aware of the various alternatives to restraint and how to apply them. Because standard professional training programs provide relatively little material on restraint alternatives, healthcare organizations usually must fill in this gap on their own. A healthcare organization should include information about available alternatives to restraint in its formal orientation procedures and regular inservice training.

Increase activities

Behavioral healthcare organizations can often eliminate the need for restraining

Figure 4.1 **Some Frequently Used Restraint Alternatives**

The following represent just a small sample of measures that have been used successfully to avoid restraint use.

Measures to reduce falls and wandering

- Orient new patients to the geography and rules of the facility.
- Pay close attention to physiological problems that can increase the danger of falling, such as postural hypotension, muscular weakness and diminished ability to walk.
- Evaluate medications to reduce the possibility of side effects, such as hypotension, poor balance, and physical weakness.
- Redesign clinical areas to reduce slippery floors, poorly lighted areas, unstable furniture, areas hidden from nursing observation, distant rest rooms, and poor nurse-patient communication systems.
- Provide such guides as signs, diagrams, and large symbols to reduce the risk of patients' getting lost and wandering.

Measures to reduce the danger of disturbing sutures, tubes, and lines

- Ask family members to sit with patients for as many hours as possible, particularly during the times when the patient seems most inclined to wander or to disturb sutures, tubes, lines, etc.
- Consider asking patients who can legally do so to accept restraint-like measures voluntarily.
- Remove tubes and lines as quickly as possible, even if there is some risk of having to reinsert them.
- Offer distracting activities such as telephone access, television programs, games, reading matter, etc.

Figure 4.1 **Some Frequently Used Restraint Alternatives (cont.)**

Measures in behavioral healthcare facilities

- Educate family members about the reasons restraint is used, the means by which restraint can be avoided, and the roles they can play in helping their relative avoid the need for restraint.
- Educate patients who are at risk for restraint regarding behavior that might trigger restraint use, available restraint alternatives to use if the patient is experiencing difficulty, and behavior that might lead to release from restraint if restraint becomes necessary.
- Unobtrusively identify patients who are at high risk for restraint so that nursing staff can increase observation and preventive efforts.
- Carefully observe patient groups to detect early stages of aggression, and intervene before aggression leads to physical conflict.
- Increase emphasis on patient-staff interaction, such as encouraging staff to do paperwork in areas in which they can observe and interact with patients.

patients who tend to wander by giving the patients activities, such as games or arts and crafts projects, to occupy their time and to motivate them to stay in one place. Such activities might even be organized by volunteers or family members—reducing the amount of staff time required for this treatment alternative.

Likewise, in a general hospital where the primary use of restraint is to prevent patients from removing tubes and dressings, adding distractions that divert patients' attention from their discomfort, and decrease the need for restraint for at least part of the day, can help. For example, a hospital might consider increasing the number of television channels, the emphasis on activities or recreation therapies, and family or volunteer visits.

Consider manipulating the design and elements of patient care settings

The physical design of a healthcare facility can strongly influence the frequency of restraint use. Therefore, healthcare organizations should make every effort to make the setup of patient care settings most conducive to avoiding the need for restraint. If staff can easily observe all areas where patients congregate during the day in a psychiatric hospital, for example, restraint is less likely to be necessary, since staff can intervene in the early stages of any negative situation that seems likely to escalate. A facility that has many hidden areas, on the other hand, has to compensate by stationing staff in scattered locations—thereby increasing the need for more staff—or face an increased risk of harm to patients and others.

Mechanical devices

The use of certain mechanical devices can provide an alternative to restraint. There are various types of alarms, for example, that alert nursing staff when a patient gets out of a chair or bed or walks out a door. These devices are particularly useful for monitoring patients who are at risk of wandering or falling when they get out of their rooms, and often they eliminate the need for restraint. Nursing call buttons or other communication devices are also effective because they keep patients from getting up and walking to request assistance.

Consider changing treatment approaches

By changing the pattern or frequency of certain treatment approaches, an organization might be able to avoid the use of restraint, or at least limit the time that certain patients must be restrained. For example, an organization should consider using nasogastric tubes or intravenous lines intermittently, when feasible. Such a change might eliminate the need for restraining patients with tubes and lines in place, or will at least significantly reduce the amount of time patients must be restrained. Although it is uncomfortable for patients and time-consuming for staff, removing and replacing tubes and lines is usually a better alternative than risking psychological and physical damage to patients as the result of prolonged restraint.

Pay careful attention to safety of the environment

By paying careful attention to the elimination of safety risks, organizations might be able to decrease or even eliminate the need for restraint on patients who are at a high risk of falling. For example, organizations should

- eliminate slippery floors;

- eliminate obstructed or dark areas;
- eliminate beds, couches, and chairs that are too high;
- place patients who tend to fall in beds that are close to the floor;
- use chairs that are stable, easy to get out of, and comfortable;
- provide patients who tend to get confused at night and are in danger of falling with easy access to call signals, and place such patients close to a nurses' station; and
- add such safety enhancements as better night lighting.

Detect and avoid behavioral triggers

When root-cause analysis (or intensive assessment) is used to examine each restraint episode or statistics regarding the facility's restraint use in general, it might become obvious that certain kinds of events often precede the need for restraint. These events should be considered as possible triggers for the behavior that requires restraint use. This information can be useful in reducing the frequency of restraint use for particular patients or within the facility as a whole. (Therefore, this approach is useful whether the facility is doing case-by-case review or statistical analyses.)

For example, when staff in a behavioral healthcare facility look at what is going on immediately before a number of restraint episodes, it appears that restraint tends to be used at patient mealtimes. On first examination, this is puzzling. Further examination of the events at mealtimes, however, shows that restraint is used when meals are served late and patients are still waiting to eat. At these times, patients are not scheduled for any other activity and are milling around anxious to begin eating. Furthermore, staffing at these times is light because some staff members have taken a break to eat their own meals. Conflicts break out among patients, and staff have difficulty seeing the confrontations develop and intervening. Staff have relatively few alternatives to restraint available to get patients under control at such times.

In another example, in an acute care hospital, statistical analysis shows that there is higher frequency of restraint use in general medical and surgical units than in intensive care units. This is surprising because obviously, patients in intensive care units are more likely to have lines and tubes inserted or to be on ventilators than patients in general units. A task force is assigned to investigate this and do a root-cause analysis, with the hope that the analysis will suggest some steps that can be taken to reduce the frequency of restraint use. The task force finds that nursing personnel in intensive care units are receiving more and better inservice training on restraint alternatives than nursing personnel in general units. The obvious step, then, is to increase the training for personnel in the general units.

Therapeutic holding

Therapeutic holding is a behavioral healthcare term that is used in two ways:

1. Therapeutic holding of patients who are young children refers to when a single staff member hugs the patient tightly and perhaps lifts the patient off the ground to get a temper tantrum or similar outburst under control. This procedure keeps the child from striking out or running away, while at the same time physically comforts the child. Because of the difference in size and strength between the patient and the staff member, this procedure can be done without any danger. Furthermore, it would be highly questionable to use mechanical restraint devices with a small child.

2. For older and larger patients, the term *therapeutic holding* is usually used to describe the process of grappling with a patient to get the patient under control to enable staff to apply mechanical restraints. Sometimes, however, the intention is not even to use mechanical restraints, but to control the patient's movements by means of the physical force staff exert by holding the patients limbs or entire body (some facilities term this procedure *physical restraint,* in contrast to *mechanical restraint,* which uses devices).

Some experts feel that therapeutic holding is more humane, less frightening, and less impersonal than the use of mechanical restraints and, therefore, consider it a less-restrictive alternative to mechanical restraint.

The JCAHO is vague on how to treat therapeutic holding. The introductory statement to the JCAHO standards on restraint and seclusion makes it clear that it views therapeutic holding differently than mechanical restraint. But the statement doesn't elaborate on how therapeutic holding should be treated. Some experts believe that the standards do not cover therapeutic holding in any way. Others interpret the statement to mean that if therapeutic holding is used less than 15 minutes, it does not qualify as restraint under the standards, but if it used longer than 15 minutes, it is considered restraint. It is quite likely that the JCAHO will soon deal with and clarify this confusion. Regardless, our recommendation is to treat therapeutic holding of patients larger than small children as even more dangerous than mechanical restraint.

There are several reasons for this increased danger.

- First and foremost is the increased likelihood of injury to patients and staff because of prolonged physical contact versus impersonal mechanical restraint.

- Second is the element of a physical contest that is introduced when an upset patient is, in effect, challenged by a group of staff, and the staff are challenged by the patient. There is too much temptation in such a situation to see who will "win" the wrestling contest, and to throw caution to the winds in doing so. In the heat of the moment, staff might use techniques to overpower the patient that at the same time cause injury.

- Third is the loss of the quieting effect of mechanical restraint. When mechanical restraint is applied and the patient is left alone in a room with nobody to impress or struggle against, the result is often recovery of control or even sleepiness.

Therapeutic holding—except as a means of getting a patient into mechanical restraint— should be used only on small children and by a single, trained staff member. Good risk management suggests that organizations should treat the use of holding—more than briefly as a step toward applying mechanical restraint—exactly the same way as they treat physical restraint, regarding the need for an order; concern for protection of patients' rights, dignity, and well-being; and documentation. Even when holding is used on a small child easily controlled by one person, it is a good idea to require two staff members to be involved—one to do the holding and the other to observe and document.

Seclusion and restraint; what is the difference?

While physical restraint and seclusion share many similarities, there are special issues organizations should consider when using seclusion.

Seclusion is used only in behavioral healthcare settings. It is usually considered to be less restrictive and less stressful for patients than restraint. Therefore, some facilities treat seclusion as a less-restrictive alternative to restraint. Other facilities classify restraint and seclusion as equally restrictive. It is common for organizations to prefer using one to the other and to use the one that isn't preferred hardly at all. JCAHO standards treat restraint and seclusion in the same way and make no distinction, except that the medical and surgical standards do not provide for use of seclusion (see Chapters 5 and 6 for more specific discussion regarding JCAHO standards).

Time out as an alternative to seclusion

A common alternative to seclusion is to request that a patient voluntarily leave the patient group—referred to as *time out*. A patient in time out might be asked to go to his or her room or a relatively quiet area of the unit. Or a patient might even go to the seclusion room for a time out, but since the room is kept unlocked and the patient is free to leave, the situation is significantly different than actual seclusion. Although one of the purposes of time out is for the patient to be alone, staff should still observe a patient in time out for safety reasons.

What to do when you *must* apply restraint

Provide patient and family education

Educating patients about the need for restraint, the process used to apply restraint, and the criteria necessary for release from restraint not only meets JCAHO requirements but also generally tends to make the whole restraint process less traumatic for patients. Patient education often shortens the time that patients are in restraint and might even eliminate the need for restraint in some cases. Effective education can also convince a patient to accept a necessary restriction voluntarily, thus eliminating the episode from being considered restraint (see Chapter 1 for more information on patient consent).

Educating patients' families about restraint can also have positive effects. (An adult patient has the right to prevent the provision of medical information to a family member, however, unless the family member has legal status as a guardian or equivalent.) Family members might help to educate patients when patients have difficulty absorbing information from staff, for instance, and might also be able to assist staff in reducing the negative effects of restraint or developing and maintaining alternatives to it, such as familial visits, which provide a distraction from the restraint, or reminding the patient of the behavior necessary to terminate restraint. Close friends can also carry out the same functions as family members, provided patients consent to it.

What to do when you *must* apply seclusion

How to safety-proof walls, ceilings, windows, and doors

A good way to evaluate a room used for seclusion is to ask the question: "How might a patient deliberately or accidentally injure himself or herself in this room?" An organization should remember that some of the individuals who will be secluded will either attempt to hurt themselves or have extremely limited judgment.

The walls of a seclusion room should be made of material that is least likely to injure patients who attempt to scratch themselves or pound their bodies against the walls. Walls should be made of a firm, smooth material and covered with paint that resists scratching and writing, and should not contain electrical or other types of outlets. Organizations might even consider designing "padded cells"—rooms whose walls are covered with padding—for patients who might attempt to harm themselves. Padded cells are relatively rare, but are effective at protecting patients (as long as the patients do not succeed in tearing the padding).

The ceiling should be high enough so even the tallest patients cannot reach it when they jump. A ceiling should not have any protruding devices, and lights should be recessed and covered with fine mesh or plastic, so patients can't hang themselves or break the bulbs.

If there is a window in a room used for seclusion, it should be made of shatter-resistant glass or plastic or be covered by an impenetrable screen. When a window is covered on the inside by a grill or grid, its screening should be fine enough that it is impossible to push even a small object through the screen. And if a window is operable, its control should either be outside the room or it should require a separate wrench or similar tool. Generally, a window should be kept closed so that room temperature is kept at a stable, cool but comfortable temperature (as noted in Chapter 3, patients in seclusion might overheat and possibly become dehydrated from struggling before or during seclusion).

The door to a seclusion room should be

- strong enough to withstand repeated, forceful kicks without bending or breaking;
- able to be locked from the outside only (although when a patient is inside, it is preferable to keep the door closed with a nonlocking bolt for easy opening);
- kept locked when there is no patient inside to prevent unauthorized individuals from entering; and
- smooth on the inside (like the material used for the walls).

In addition, if the door has a window to allow patient observation, the window should be safety-proofed (as described above) and should permit observation of every part of the inside of the room. If a room's design does not permit observation of all corners from the observation window, it should be equipped with a metal mirror that reveals all parts of the room but that is not accessible to secluded patients (for instance, a mirror mounted high on a wall or on the ceiling).

Seclusion rooms do not usually contain furniture—primarily because of the possibility that patients might break the furniture and use the parts as weapons. If an organization considers including beds in its seclusion rooms, as some organizations do, it should make sure that the beds are strong and heavy enough that they cannot be broken or moved. Unbreakable, heavy beds might still be dangerous because they might allow patients to reach the ceiling or leap from a height. An organization should consider equipping seclusion rooms with mats for sleeping instead.

Observe secluded patients

Many hospitals require staff to observe secluded patients only every 15 minutes. Others have staff members continually observe secluded patients via closed-circuit TV—often at a location removed from the seclusion room. But these setups are dangerous because patients can harm themselves when they are not being observed and staff will probably not be able to intervene as quickly as possible when patients get into trouble. The safest way to implement seclusion is to have a staff member situated right outside the seclusion room door, constantly observing the patient.

Some facilities even place an observer directly in the seclusion room with the patient, which provides immediate access and fosters staff-patient communication. But there are two drawbacks to this strategy: (1) some mentally ill patients might attempt to overcome a solo staff observer; and (2) the purpose of seclusion for some patients is to isolate them and eliminate all extraneous stimulation, so a staff member's presence might be distracting and defeats the purpose of seclusion for such patients.

Make communication easy

Secluded patients should be able to easily communicate with staff, although one of the main reasons for seclusion is to isolate them and provide them with the opportunity to calm down. Therefore, in an ideal situation, staff should be able to hear a patient but the patient should not be able to see staff members. Some organizations use microphone-speaker systems in seclusion rooms to permit two-way communication and enable staff to hear what is happening in the room. Other facilities place call buttons in seclusion rooms. All organizations should place call buttons outside seclusion rooms for staff observers to use in case there is an emergency in the seclusion room and additional staff are needed immediately.

All communication between a secluded patient and staff, other patients, and visitors should be controlled—not only for therapeutic reasons but also to protect the patient's confidentiality and privacy. No other patients should be able to see, hear, or communicate with a secluded patient. In many organizations, a seclusion room is in an entirely separate area of the facility that can be locked to prevent unauthorized access.

Carefully choose the location of seclusion rooms

The location of seclusion rooms is as important as their design. A seclusion room should, for example,

- be close to where additional help is immediately available—usually the nurses' station;
- be protected from the view of patients and visitors;
- be far enough away that other patients and visitors are not able to hear patient shouts or pounding;
- have air conditioning and heating ducts, since the room needs to be kept at a comfortable temperature; and
- be close to a toilet, since it is best to move a patient who has to go to the toilet out of the room, but not from the general area.

Many seclusion rooms are part of a locked suite that includes a small room containing a sink and a toilet. If such as suite is easily accessible from the nurses' station, then it meets many of the location requirements for seclusion rooms. Such a suite should have two doors—one connecting with the nurses' station and the other to the hall or corridor.

Staff training

Most organizations that use seclusion combine training on seclusion application with training on restraint application. Although there is a considerable amount of overlap between the skills required for restraint and those for seclusion, there are differences that must be covered in training.

How to make clinical decisions

Although ultimate responsibility for decisions involving restraint or seclusion rests with physicians, nursing staff often make initial, emergency decisions. Therefore, staff training should cover how to make clinical decisions regarding when and what type of restraint or seclusion is appropriate.

Staff should be able to recognize when seclusion is more appropriate than restraint, since it is generally considered a less restrictive procedure than restraint and is, therefore, used for less disturbed patients. Because secluded patients can seriously harm themselves—by banging their heads against the wall, scratching at their skin, or even hanging themselves—it is critical that staff be trained to master the clinical skill of determining whether a patient is safe for seclusion and does not need restraint. In addition, staff should also be trained to know when restraint and seclusion should be combined. Some hospitals use the term *restraint plus seclusion* to describe a situation in which a restrained patient is locked in a room alone.

How to apply safety measures

Staff should also be trained on what preparatory procedures—particularly safety measures—they must carry out before secluding a patient. Since secluded patients might attempt to harm themselves, especially if they possess dangerous objects, staff need to know what items are inappropriate, what type of clothing is unsafe, and how to make sure that they don't possess any dangerous items.

How to evaluate if patients should be released from seclusion

Staff must learn how to determine whether a patient can be released from seclusion. Furthermore, since seclusion is used mainly in behavioral healthcare facilities—where the JCAHO standards limit the length of seclusion orders to four hours but allow nursing and other personnel to extend the orders—staff need training on how to evaluate patients to determine whether to extend seclusion orders. Even if a facility uses a checklist to evaluate secluded patients, staff require training to use it.

How to observe and interact with secluded patients

Staff members who observe and communicate with secluded patients should be trained to do so. Since most organizations use a checklist to guide the observation of patients in seclusion, staff should be shown how to complete it. They should also be trained to determine how to respond to dangerous behaviors that secluded patients might exhibit. Finally, staff should be able to decide when communication with secluded patients is therapeutic and when it is not.

Note: Figure 4.2 summarizes and describes the JCAHO's expectations concerning staff competence in applying restraint and seclusion.

Figure 4.2 Required Levels of Competence for Staff Involved in Applying Restraint or Seclusion

The following JCAHO standards regarding the competence of staff who use restraint or seclusion are in the JCAHO hospital standards for behavioral health-care settings (TX 7.1 through TX.7.1.3.2). The hospital standards for medical and surgical settings (TX.7.5 through TX.7.5.5) do not contain any references to staff training. Good risk management and clinical care, however, require that these standards (and arguably even additional requirements) be followed in any setting in which restraint is used.

The 1999 standards for behavioral health care (i.e., freestanding behavioral health-care organizations) are the ones applicable to hospitals before 1999 and are discussed on page 58 of the first edition of this book. Please contact the publisher of this book, Opus Communications, for more information.

TX.7.1.1.3: [Leaders have responsibility for] Staff orientation and education creating a culture emphasizing prevention and appropriate use and encouraging alternatives.
This standard focuses on staff attitudes and habits (i.e., culture), rather than any technical aspects of using restraint. This standard recognizes what now seems to be professional consensus that appropriateness and frequency of restraint use are strongly influenced by values and customs in each institution. JCAHO expects leaders to evaluate these values and customs and change them, if necessary.

TX.7.1.3.1.2: Restraint or seclusion use is based on the assessed needs of the patient.
The intent statement of this standard makes clear that one essential element of assessment is appropriate training and skill of those who are authorized to initiate emergency use of restraint in the absence of a licensed, independent practitioner. This group typically comprises registered nurses, although in some organizations the group is restricted to nurse supervisors. In any case, these individuals should receive training on recognizing the need for restraint initiation and on the steps to take as restraint is carried out.

TX.7.1.3.1.4: Restraint or seclusion is used correctly by competent, trained staff.
The intent statement of this standard explains that safe and effective use of restraint depends on having staff who are competent in the necessary skills. Skills are separated into two groups: (1) initiation and termination; and (2) application and removal. The first group presumably is limited to supervisory or more experienced personnel who are trained in assessment of patients (and documentation of assessment). The second group—which is likely to be far larger and to include the members of the first group—is trained in actual hands-on techniques.

The statement mentions, and organizations should therefore consider: frequent inservice training; competence to use the restraint devices involved; and including the experiences of patients who have undergone restraint in staff training.

Chapter Five

Overview of the New JCAHO Standards and Survey Process

What prompted the 1999 restraint standards changes?

On July 1, 1996, a revised set of JCAHO standards concerning restraint and seclusion went into effect for hospitals, ambulatory care facilities, and behavioral healthcare facilities. These standards were intended to help to meet two goals: (1) to establish a single set of standards for all JCAHO accreditation programs (the 1996 long-term care and home care restraint standards differed somewhat, but shared the same philosophical emphasis); and (2) to definitively label restraint and seclusion as high-risk procedures that require careful scrutiny and reduced use. (The long-term care standards are more influenced by the philosophy of complete restraint elimination.)

The 1996 standards created a number of problems, however, particularly in acute-care, general hospitals. The total percentages of facilities that received Type I recommendations between 1996 through 1998 on restraint-related standards across the JCAHO accreditation programs was higher than in any other area. This makes the restraint standards the most problematic standards across all JCAHO manuals, and it suggests that even leading, heavily staffed hospitals have difficulty in complying.

In response to the problems, the JCAHO carried out a study in the fall of 1997 that included public hearings in several locations throughout the United States. Representatives from hospitals and other healthcare facilities, as well as representatives from professional organizations, argued for revised JCAHO standards.

At the same time, numerous studies and articles published in professional journals firmly established the negative aspects of restraint use. In addition, the JCAHO's new program of monitoring "sentinel events"—adverse occurrences that result in patient death or serious injury—in accredited organizations revealed that by the end of 1998, restraint-related incidents composed a significant portion of the reported sentinel events.

Another indication of the dangers of restraint use was a series of newspaper articles in the *Hartford Courant* that reported and analyzed over 100 recent restraint-related deaths in behavioral healthcare facilities. In response to these articles, the National Alliance for the Mentally Ill (NAMI), a national advocacy group, began a campaign to establish federally enforced standards for restraint use. As a result, in early 1999, federal legislation was introduced concerning restraint, a congressional request was made to the Government Accounting Office for an investigation into restraint practices, and Congress was considering holding hearings on the issue.

In response to the hearings and its findings, the JCAHO developed a new set of 1999 restraint and seclusion standards. The JCAHO was able to analyze the sentinel event data to determine trends and offer suggestions for preventing adverse outcomes related to restraint. These new standards took effect January 1, 1999, in the accreditation programs for hospitals and ambulatory care facilities (the JCAHO did not change its standards from 1996 for the behavioral healthcare, long-term care, and home care accreditation programs, however, as discussed below).

1999 standards present problems

But the 1999 changes have failed to simplify matters; they are complex and confusing. Unlike the 1996 standards, the 1999 standards for hospitals are sharply separated between standards that are applicable to general (medical and surgical) acute care and standards that are applicable to behavioral health care. Eight of the 29 restraint-related standards in the *1999 Comprehensive Accreditation Manual for Hospitals (CAMH)* apply to general acute care in hospitals and ambulatory care facilities, while 21 are specific to behavioral healthcare units within general hospitals and to freestanding psychiatric hospitals. While there was one set of restraint standards in three accreditation manuals from 1996 to 1999, since July 1, 1999, there are two sets in the *CAMH*, a new single set in the *1999 Comprehensive Accreditation Manual for Ambulatory Care (CAMAC)*, and the old 1996 standards in the *1999 Comprehensive Accreditation Manual for Behavioral Health Care (CAMBHC)*. (See Figure 5.1 for a summary of which JCAHO standards apply to specific healthcare settings.)

In addition, while all of the 1996 standards applied to all accreditation programs—hospitals, ambulatory care, and behavioral health care—the 1999 standards, in contrast, are not uniform across the accreditation programs. The *CAMBHC* still contains the 1996 standards, and the only new standards that the *CAMAC* contains are the same eight new standards for general acute care that are in the *1999 CAMH*.

To complicate matters even more, as of July 1999 the JCAHO has still not updated some of its materials to reflect the 1999 changes. For example, although the current *automated* version of the *CAMAC* (ambulatory care) is marked 1998–1999, it still contains the 1996 standards, not the eight new 1999 standards. And the 1999 *CAMBHC* (behavioral health care) still includes four standards dealing with the use of protocols to authorize restraint, even though the use of protocols is not permitted in behavioral healthcare settings.

What this chapter covers

This chapter explores the new 1999 JCAHO standards and survey process primarily from a hospital-based viewpoint. But readers from other types of facilities will find the discussion equally relevant because many of the behavioral health care and ambulatory care restraint standards are the same as the hospital standards, just with different standard numbers.

In many instances, for the sake of simplicity, the term *restraint* in this chapter refers to both restraint and seclusion. Almost every behavioral health care restraint standard applies equally to seclusion. When necessary, this chapter discusses seclusion separately. As mentioned in Chapter 1, the new restraint standards do not apply to what is called *chemical restraint*—the use of sedative or tranquilizing drugs. As with physical restraint and seclusion, the JCAHO is also concerned with the negative effects of chemical restraint, but it covers the use of chemical restraint under the standards relating to medication use in the *Care of the Patient (TX), Patient*

Figure 5.1 Which Set of Restraint Standards Applies to Each Setting?

Setting	Applicable Accreditation Manual and Standards
Hospital	
Freestanding psychiatric hospital Psychiatric unit in general hospital Medical or surgical patient transferred for psychiatric care	Hospital Manual, Behavioral Healthcare Standards (TX.7.1–TX.7.1.3.2)
Emergency room Psychiatric patient transferred for medical or surgical care All other parts of hospital	Hospital Manual, Medical/Surgical Standards (TX.7.5–TX.7.5.5)
Hospital-owned behavioral residential treatment center	Behavioral Health Care Manual (TX.3.1–TX.3.1.3.3)
Hospital-owned long-term care facility	Long-term care facilities—regardless of ownership, affiliation, or location—are subject to standards TX.8 through TX.8.1 in the accreditation manual for long-term care. These standards differ from the standards discussed in this book.
Ambulatory care	
Hospital-owned facility	Hospital Manual, Medical/Surgical Standards (TX.7.5–TX.7.5.5)
Freestanding facility	Ambulatory Manual (TX.7–TX.7.5)
Behavioral healthcare facility (regardless of ownership)	Behavioral Health Care Manual (TX.3.1–TX.3.1.3.3)
Behavioral residential facility (not a hospital)	Behavioral Health Care Manual (TX.3.1–TX.3.1.3.3)

Rights and Organization Ethics (RI), and *Leadership (LD)* chapters of its accreditation manuals.

Restraint standards are somewhat prescriptive

Today, most of the JCAHO's standards and intent statements are generally nonprescriptive, allowing hospitals flexibility to comply in a way that best fits their needs. Rather than dictating a course of action, surveyors are likely to ask about a hospital's policy and assess whether staff are following that policy. Before 1996, the sole JCAHO standard in the *CAMH* relating to restraint, TX.7.1, was no exception. It was nonprescriptive, and it allowed individual organizations to settle many details regarding restraint use.

But many of the 1996 and new 1999 restraint standards are a modest deviation from this nonprescriptive approach. With the current restraint standards, many common clinical practices have become requirements, and there are a small number of highly specific requirements in the intent statements of some restraint standards that are vital to an organization's overall score. For example, the standards require healthcare organizations and professionals to consider and document their reasons for using restraint for every restraint episode. Physicians who are accustomed to including restraint as part of routine orders, or who tend to write and renew orders for restraint use that continue for many days, must now rethink these practices. The standards also now require staff training in several aspects of restraint use; restraint is no longer considered a procedure with which every healthcare professional is familiar simply by virtue of being a healthcare professional.

Furthermore, even though many restraint standards are still generally nonprescriptive, (much of a hospital's accreditation score is based on compliance with its own policies and procedures), and even though many of the discussions and specific examples on how to comply with the restraint standards in the *CAMH* are guidelines and are not binding in any way, the JCAHO is now specific in how it expects hospitals to comply. That is, the JCAHO no longer allows hospitals to simply incorporate the standards verbatim into their policies; it now expects each hospital to develop its own policies that detail how the hospital interprets and fulfills these standards within its unique circumstances.

A summary of the significant themes and requirements

Generally, the 1996 and new 1999 JCAHO restraint standards do not represent a change in direction or an introduction of new concepts. Most of the themes embedded in the new standards were explicit or implied in the old, all-encompassing TX.7.1 restraint standard and intent statement. There is little, if anything, in the new standards that should surprise experienced healthcare personnel.

What might be surprising, however, is the intensity of attention the JCAHO now expects healthcare organizations to give to restraint use. The following eight points summarize the major themes and expectations of the JCAHO's new restraint standards (Chapter 6 provides specific information on each individual standard).

- **Have a plan, policies, and procedures devoted to restraint:** The JCAHO now requires hospitals to have a plan and a set of policies and procedures that cover a variety of aspects of restraint use. These items might be contained in other documents—rather than individual restraint-only documents—as long as they specifically cover restraint-related areas in detail.

- **Use restraint only when necessary:** The JCAHO now considers restraint a high-risk procedure that should be used only when absolutely necessary—never routinely or without careful, documented consideration. Facilities must demonstrate an effort to reduce the frequency of restraint use.

- **Justify restraint use:** As mentioned above, the JCAHO requires organizations to justify—or explain—every episode of restraint. The justification for every restraint episode should comply with hospital policy requirements. In addition, staff should document the justification in the patient's medical record and include a description of the less restrictive alternatives that staff attempted but that failed to control the problematic behavior.

- **Assess before applying restraint:** The JCAHO now requires hospitals to assess patients who might require restraint and to document the findings of the assessment before applying restraint. An assessment must consider the needs and goals of the patient's treatment. Even an emergency use of restraint should involve an assessment. (Although an emergency assessment, of course, should be documented after the situation is under control.)

- **Train staff and evaluate competency:** The JCAHO requires that all staff involved in initiating, applying, and terminating restraint should be appropriately trained and demonstrate competency in the roles they play in restraint use. Certain staff members with additional authority and responsibility, such as registered nurses and nursing managers, should be specially trained and tested to perform such tasks as directing application of emergency restraint or using a nursing protocol to authorize restraint.

- **Measure, assess, and improve restraint use:** The new standards require hospitals to improve performance in relation to restraint use. They must measure and assess restraint use and demonstrate that they implement efforts to reduce the frequency of it.

- **Educate patients and families:** The standards applicable to behavioral healthcare settings require hospitals and other behavioral healthcare facilities to educate patients who are candidates for restraint or who are already in restraint. Presumably, the information should describe measures that the patient can take to prevent or end restraint use. When educating patients is not possible, such as when they are not competent to make decisions, hospitals should educate family members, when appropriate, specifically in ways they can help to avoid the need for restraint. Patient and family education in restraint in acute care settings remains a leadership responsibility, but it is no longer specifically required by a restraint standard, although it is mentioned in an intent statement. (See Chapter 4, pp. 79-80, for more information on patient and family education and related issues, such as patient consent and family involvement in applying alternatives to restraint.)

- **Protect patient rights, dignity, and well-being:** The new standards require hospitals to protect the rights, dignity, and physical and mental well-being of restrained patients. Before the new standards, this obvious expectation was taken for granted.

Figure 5.2 presents a summary of the JCAHO's major issues regarding restraint and seclusion and lists which standards relate to each.

Changes in the survey process

Over the past five years, the JCAHO has made major changes in its survey process. In the past, standard interpretations were almost completely subjective and varied greatly among JCAHO surveyors. Outsiders had little, if any, information on how surveyors were instructed to score standards. Contemporary surveyors, however, have information in hard copy and on laptop computers to help them interpret the standards objectively and consistently. And most of this material is available to the public in various JCAHO publications. Furthermore, while surveyors used to spend a lot of time scrutinizing hospital policies and procedures, quality assurance records, meeting minutes, and other documents, they now spend more of their time interviewing patients and staff, observing staff in action, and examining the details of the physical environment.

To assess compliance with the restraint standards, surveyors usually ask to review the charts of any patients currently in the facility who have been restrained, and they might request to interview one or more of these patients. If surveyors observe a patient in restraint, they will likely discuss the episode with staff and examine the medical record to determine whether documentation is complete and accurate.

But because some of the new restraint standards are so general, as discussed above, experts (including surveyors) sometimes disagree about the precise meaning or applicability of a standard and have no objective way to settle the disagreement. For example, standard TX.7.1.3.1.4 requires that only competent, trained staff apply restraint; but how does one determine staff competency? What is the required extent of training?

Each hospital must determine these issues for itself, and it must do so in a deliberate, planned, and systematic way. To demonstrate the forethought and resources that went into creating their policies and procedures, hospital representatives should discuss their perspective on the meaning of particular standards with surveyors and show surveyors relevant hospital documents. Furthermore, a hospital

Figure 5.2 Primary JCAHO Issues and Related Standards

Issue	Related Standards
Justification	TX.7.1 TX.7.1.1 TX.7.5 TX.7.5.3.2
Patient assessment	TX.7.1.1.5 TX.7.1.3 TX.7.1.3.1.2 TX.7.5.2
Prevention of use	TX.7.1.1.3 TX.7.1.1.5 TX.7.1.1.7
Policies & procedures	TX.7.1.1.1 TX.7.1.3 TX.7.5.2
Human resource planning	TX.7.1.1.2
Human resource orientation & education	TX.7.1.1.3
Human resource competence	TX.7.1.3.1.4
Patient & family education	TX.7.1.1.4
Care plan	TX.7.1.1.6
Performance improvement	TX.7.1.2 TX.7.5.1
Patient rights	TX.7.1.3.1.1 TX.7.5.2 Intent
Protocol use	TX.7.5.3 TX.7.5.3.2
Documentation	TX.7.1.3.2 TX.7.5.5
Appropriate orders	TX.7.1.3.1 TX.7.1.3.1.7 TX.7.5.3.1

should make sure its medical staff and other appropriate bodies approve its restraint policies and procedures, and it should show surveyors that it has done so. This high-level approval will likely avoid having to debate the question of whether a department's policy is clinically appropriate with a surveyor who might disagree with what an individual department head has determined.

Organizations must continually collect information regarding the JCAHO's survey process, which is constantly evolving. Surveyors accumulate experience evaluating particular standards and report their findings and difficulties to JCAHO headquarters. The JCAHO uses this feedback to make adjustments to the survey process. The way in which surveyors assess compliance with the 1999 restraint standards will almost certainly evolve. Information on current surveyor practices can usually be found in the newsletters of Opus Communications and several Internet sources (contact Opus Communications for more information).

The survey agenda

Hospital survey agendas are set well in advance through a consultation between the hospital and the JCAHO central office. Survey agendas for other JCAHO accreditation programs are usually established through a discussion between a surveyor and a representative of the surveyed organization.

Under the pre-1996 restraint standard (TX.7.1), surveyors evaluated restraint informally and at no set time. Restraint was just one of many issues, and not the most important issue. Today, however, there is a heavy emphasis on restraint use in several survey events. There is no single event in the survey agenda that is devoted to restraint; surveyors evaluate compliance with the restraint standards through a number of agenda events that cover other issues in addition to restraint, as summarized below.

Document Review Session

Surveyors examine JCAHO-required documents in this initial phase of the survey. (Before its survey, a healthcare organization receives a list of documents that the JCAHO requires it to make available to surveyors.) In addition to these required documents, a healthcare organization has the opportunity to show surveyors additional restraint-related documents that contribute important information.

Restraint-related documents that are appropriate for this session (some are required; others are helpful if a hospital has them) include the following. Although the presence or absence—as well as the quality—of relevant documents influences the scoring of any restraint standard, some specific restraint standards require certain documents. These standards are indicated in parentheses following the appropriate documents. (All standards numbers here and below are from the *CAMH*; underlined standard numbers refer to behavioral health units in hospitals, while standard numbers that are not underlined refer to medical/surgical care.)

- medical staff bylaws;
- medical staff rules and regulations;
- relevant plans, policies, and statements of priorities (TX.7.1.1.1 and TX.7.5.2);
- human resource plans (TX.7.1.1.2);
- policies and procedures (TX.7.1.3 and TX.7.5.2);
- clinical protocols (TX.7.5.3.2);
- training curricula;
- resource allocation plans;
- lists of qualified personnel and criteria used to assess qualification;
- performance improvement (PI) data measurements and assessments; and
- PI reports.

A healthcare organization should consider placing all restraint-related documents for this session in a separate folder or binder or preparing an index that shows the locations of the documents to provide surveyors with easy access to them.

Closed Medical Record Review (part of the Medical Record Interview)
During this session, hospital staff—under the direction of surveyors—examine closed medical records. (In small hospitals, staff are asked to review designated closed records before the survey and report their findings during the Medical Record Interview.)

Surveyors request that some of the records contain documentation of restraint or seclusion episodes to review whether they include the following. The standard numbers that apply to each item are in parentheses. (As above, all standards are from the *CAMH*; underlined standard numbers refer to behavioral health units in hospitals, while standard numbers that are not underlined refer to medical/surgical care.) [1]

- licensed independent practitioner orders for restraint (TX.7.1.3.2.7, TX.7.5.3, and TX.7.5.3.1);
- written time limits as part of restraint orders (TX.7.1.3.2.8);
- documentation that restraint episodes complied with JCAHO standards (particularly TX.7.1.3.3) and hospital bylaws, rules and regulations, policies, and procedures (TX.7.5.3 and TX.7.5.3.1);
- evidence that restrained patients were assessed prior to initiation of restraint and were regularly observed while in restraint (TX.7.1.1.5, TX.7.1.3.2.2, and TX.7.5.3);
- evidence that patients' rights, dignity, and privacy were protected (TX.7.1.3.2.1);
- documentation showing attention to patient needs (TX.7.1.3.2.6 and TX.7.5.4);

1 *Some items that are mentioned in the TX.7.5 set of standards (medical and surgical care) do not appear here because the list here is taken from the JCAHO form that is used to evaluate records in the Closed Medical Record Review session. The form ignores issues such as the requirement that restraint orders in medical and surgical facilities be limited to 24 hours (TX.7.5.3.1 Intent).*

- appropriate renewal or continuation of restraint orders (TX.7.1.3.2.8); and
- documentation showing that any initiation of restraint under a protocol meets clinical justification requirements (TX.7.5.3.2).

Open Medical Record Review

Surveyors are likely to request the medical records of patients who are or were restrained during their visits to patient care units. Surveyors examine the records for evidence of compliance with JCAHO and hospital-specific requirements.

Surveyors combine the findings from the open and closed medical record reviews to determine scores for those restraint standards that are scored based on the percentage of compliant records (TX.7.1.3.1.7, TX.7.1.3.1.8, TX.7.1.3.2, and TX.7.5.3). Surveyors also develop general impressions of how a hospital carries out restraint by looking at medical records in these sessions.

Survey interviews

A large proportion of staff interviews includes questions regarding restraint use. The following section describes what a hospital can expect in each of these interviews and cites related standards, where appropriate.

- **Medical Record Interview:** The Medical Record Interview focuses on the organization's own reviews of the completeness, timeliness, and quality of medical records documentation. Although there are no restraint standards that specifically relate to the Medical Record Interview, surveyors are likely to inquire about the level of attention that staff members who regularly review medical records give to restraint documentation.
- **Leadership Interview:** Surveyors will almost certainly ask one or more questions pertaining to restraint use or compliance with any of the restraint standards during the Leadership Interview. The restraint standards that deal specifically with leadership responsibilities include TX.7.1.1 (not scored), TX.7.1.1.1, TX.7.1.1.2, TX.7.1.1.3, TX.7.1.1.4, TX.7.1.1.5, TX.7.1.1.6, TX.7.1.1.7, and TX.7.5.

- **Medical Staff Leadership Interview:** In a hospital survey, the physician surveyor is concerned with the medical staff's involvement in developing and executing the hospital's approach to restraint. Although the surveyor might ask questions regarding a variety of aspects of restraint use or any of the restraint standards, he or she is likely to focus on the following standards that generally relate to medical staff responsibilities: TX.7.1.3.1.1, TX.7.1.3.2, TX.7.1.3.2.7, and TX.7.1.3.2.8. For medical/surgical areas, the principle standard relating to medical staff responsibilities is TX.7.5, which concerns leadership responsibilities.

- **Nursing Leadership Interview:** Nurses play a major role in most aspects of restraint use. Therefore, they are generally responsible for, and are likely to be asked questions regarding, the following standards TX.7.1.3.1.4, TX.7.1.3.1.5, TX.7.1.3.1.6, and TX.7.5.4.

- **Chief Executive Officer (CEO) Interview:** The CEO does not have any specific responsibilities under the restraint standards, in contrast to the group of leaders as a whole. But because a number of the restraint standards have significant financial implications and because the CEO is responsible to the board for everything that happens in the organization, surveyors are likely to ask the CEO questions regarding (1) how much effort and resources are devoted to training staff on restraint and what indications show that these resources are sufficient, and (2) how the CEO, as the representative of the board, monitors restraint use.

- **Department Head Interview:** As a group, department heads do not have specific responsibilities relating to restraint, so surveyors are not likely to pursue the topic during this interview. Because some of the departments represented in the Department Head Interview use restraint, however, it is quite likely that surveyors will separately ask the representatives of those departments general questions regarding restraint.

- **Operative and Other Procedures Interview:** Although there are no restraint standards that apply specifically to operative and other procedures, and there are no operative and other procedures standards that deal specifically with restraint, there is still considerable overlap between the two areas in most hospitals. For example, a patient undergoing an operative or other procedure is often tied down—sometimes by all four limbs—to the operating table or treatment apparatus. While this use of ties does not necessarily fall under the restraint standards if it qualifies as an exception under hospital policy (see the discussion on opt-outs in Chapter 1, p. 37), surveyors can assume that all uses of ties constitute restraint if not otherwise stated in hospital policy. Hospital participants in this interview should be prepared to discuss whether restraint is ever used in connection with operative or other procedures and, if it is, to answer questions regarding any restraint standards.

- **Human Resources Interview:** Surveyors examine the personnel records of selected staff to determine whether the staff received appropriate orientation, periodic inservice training, and reorientation on restraint use, including the use of alternatives, preventive steps, protocols, techniques for physically controlling patients, and criteria for release from restraint. In behavioral health settings, surveyors also check whether nursing personnel records show evidence that nurses were trained in, and can demonstrate competency in, the process for extending restraint orders. The specific standards relevant to the Human Resources Interview are TX.7.1.1.2 and TX.7.1.1.3.

- **Ethics Interview:** Many of the restraint standards concern patients' rights, since restraint can be inherently demeaning and lead to loss of autonomy, dignity, and privacy (see Chapter 3 p. 56, for more discussion of this issue). Some of these standards are in the Patient Rights and Organizational Ethics chapter, including RI.1 (maintaining respect for patients), RI.1.2 (continuing care and patient participation in care), and RI.1.3.2 (maintaining patients' privacy). In addition, standard TX.7.1.3.1.1 specifically requires hospitals to protect restrained behavioral health patients' rights, dignity, and well-being. Therefore, in addition to professional and organizational ethics, surveyors ask about measures the hospital takes to protect restrained patients during the Ethics Interview.

- **Patient Care Interview:** In small-hospital surveys, a number of the traditional interviews that focus on various aspects of patient care—for example, the Operative and Other Procedures Interview and the Medication Use and Nutrition Interview—might, in the interest of saving time, be combined into one interview: the Patient Care Interview. The Patient Care Interview focuses on the hospital's execution of policies and procedures and its practical experience regarding restraint use. While the Patient Care Interview might cover any of the restraint standards, its short length of time usually restricts the depth of surveyors' questions, which cover a wide range of subjects.

- **Patient and Family Education Interview:** Education is an important element of restraint use for behavioral healthcare patients (see Chapter 4, p.79, for more discussion on patient and family education). Standard TX.7.1.1.4 requires that when a hospital uses restraint—or when there is a possibility that it might have to use restraint—it must provide the patient and, if appropriate, the patient's family members with information about the restraint procedure. In addition, standards PF.4 and PF.4.2 require that education planning include restraint, and that patients and their families have the opportunity to discuss restraint use. Surveyors evaluate a hospital's patient and family education in restraint use during this interview.

Performance Improvement (PI) Events

Because the measurement and assessment of restraint use and the steps taken to reduce it are such important hospital activities, several PI events in the survey agenda address restraint use, as discussed below.

- **Performance Improvement Overview:** A hospital should mention, at least briefly, any data and data assessment relating to restraint use and any attempts to reduce or improve restraint use during this session (TX.7.1.2, TX.7.5.1, and PI.3.1.1 [which applies to both behavioral healthcare and medical/surgical patients)]).

- **Performance Improvement Coordinating Group Interview**: Surveyors are likely to ask for information about the collection and use of data relating to restraint use during this interview (TX.7.1.2, TX.7.5.1, and PI.3.1.1 [which applies to both behavioral healthcare and medical/surgical patients]).

- **Performance Improvement Team Interview:** If a hospital has made an effort to improve restraint use through staff investigations, the hospital should have this group that carried out the investigations present its findings and recommended solutions to the surveyors.

Facility tours

Surveyors evaluate restraint use during several facility tours, as discussed below.

- **Patient Care Unit Visits:** Surveyors evaluate the hospital's performance on any of the restraint standards during patient care unit visits. On a visit to a general medical unit, for example, surveyors are likely to question how restraint is used on patients receiving intravenous medications or being treated with other types of tubes and catheters. On a visit to a psychiatric unit, surveyors will examine the seclusion room. And on a visit to any type of unit, surveyors are likely to

  - ask if there is currently a patient in restraint and, if so, ask to examine that patient's medical record and possibly interview the patient;

  - ask staff members about the hospital's restraint policies and any recent experiences the staff have had using restraint; and

  - propose a hypothetical scenario about restraint and ask staff members how they would deal with it (e.g., "If you have a patient in restraint on this unit, how do you protect the patient's rights and dignity?").

- **Imaging Services Visit:** Most radiology departments occasionally tie down patients undergoing x-rays. Unless a hospital's policies and procedures demonstrate that this use of ties does not fall under its definition of restraint, all of the JCAHO's restraint standards apply to these incidents. Even when a hospital's policies and procedures demonstrate that this use of ties does not fall under its definition of restraint, imaging services staff need to be able to discuss the applicability of the restraint standards to their department.

- **Emergency Services Visit:** Most emergency rooms use restraint fairly often—typically for psychiatric or intoxicated patients or for patients undergoing difficult procedures—if only for brief periods. Therefore, emergency room staff should be knowledgeable about the restraint standards and able to demonstrate compliance with them. (Note: The *medical/surgical* restraint standards, not the behavioral healthcare standards, apply in the emergency area.)

- **Environment of Care Tour:** One of the surveyors—usually the administrator surveyor—tours the entire facility to evaluate the hospital's compliance with the environment of care standards. During this tour, the surveyor will evaluate at least one or more seclusion rooms (if applicable) and any areas where patients are likely to be restrained. The surveyor is likely to be specifically concerned with the following areas relating to restraint use:

  – the appropriateness and adequacy of the setting to protect patients' rights, dignity, and well-being (TX.7.1.3.1.1);

  – the safety, cleanliness, and temperature of the setting (EC.4.2);

  – the design of the area (EC.4.2.1); and

  – the appropriateness and adequacy of the setting to protect patients' privacy (EC.4.3).

Contingent restraint in behavioral healthcare settings

As Chapter 2 discusses, some behavioral healthcare settings use contingent restraint or seclusion (see p. 51 for more information). These organizations should make their policies and procedures regarding contingent restraint or seclusion available to surveyors during the Document Review Session. They should also be able to answer questions regarding contingent restraint or seclusion during the surveyors' facility tour and particularly during the Open Medical Record Review session.

Because contingent restraint can be considered a clear instance of a behavior management procedure, several specific standards apply: TX.7.4, TX.7.4.1, and PI.3.1.

Some fine points on the scoring of the new standards

The JCAHO recognizes that when it revises its standards, organizations cannot make the requisite changes to their policies and procedures overnight. In looking back at compliance history, the JCAHO understands that the transition cannot be instantaneous. Immediately after standards are revised, surveyors expect only that staff and leadership are familiar with the new changes, and they evaluate the organization's compliance with the prior JCAHO standards and with the policies that were in effect before the changes. As time passes after the release of new standards, surveyors expect greater degrees of compliance with the new standards. Regarding the 1999 restraint standards, in general, surveyors now expect a healthcare organization to have a revised policy in place and to be in complete compliance with the new standards.

Some of the new restraint standards are not scored as individual standards; instead, the scores for these standards are combined with that of other standards to get a final, overall score. These situations are indicated in both the *CAMH* and in this book by the following statement: "This standard is scored at [the number of another standard]." (Figure 5.3 lists the other standards, by chapter, whose scores are influenced or determined by restraint or seclusion practices.)

Figure 5.3 **Other Hospital Standards Whose Scores Are Affected by Restraint or Seclusion Practices**

Chapter	Specific Standards*	Restraint Standards*
Management of Human Resources	HR.4 HR.4.2	TX.7.1.1.3 TX.7.1.1.3
Leadership	LD.1.1.1 LD.2.4 LD.2.5	TX.7.1.1.1 TX.7.1.1.2 TX.7.1.1.2
Assessment of Patients	PE.1.1 PE.3.1 PE.6 PE.7 PE.8	TX.7.1.1.5 TX.7.1.1.5 TX.7.1.1.5 TX.7.1.1.5 TX.7.1.1.5
Education	PF.4 PF.4.2	TX.7.1.1.4 TX.7.1.1.4
Care of Patients	TX.1 TX.1.1	TX.7.1.1.6 TX.7.1.1.6

*The chapter names and standard numbers in this table are from the *CAMH*.

Chapter Six

Individual Analyses of the New JCAHO Standards

A quick look at the new standards

Chapter 5 presented an overview of the 29 new JCAHO restraint and seclusion standards as a group. This chapter discusses each of the standards individually and in detail. Of the 29 new standards, which replace the 25 standards in the 1996 manual, 21 are specific to behavioral healthcare units or beds within general hospitals and to freestanding psychiatric hospitals (TX.7.1 through TX.7.1.2.3). These 21 standards are basically the same as 21 of the 1996 standards that applied to hospitals, behavioral healthcare, and ambulatory organizations, although they are renumbered slightly.

The remaining eight completely new standards apply to restraint use for hospital patients whose diagnoses are not primarily behavioral health–related and who are in settings that provide acute medical or surgical care: that is, hospitals, ambulatory care, and rehabilitation facilities (TX.7.5 through TX.7.5.5). These eight standards deal specifically with restraint, since seclusion is to be used only in behavioral healthcare settings. The extent of applicability of these standards varies among hospitals, since some hospitals use restraint-like procedures that the JCAHO exempts from its standards (see Chapter 1, p. 37 for a discussion of "opt-outs").

In 1996, the standards for the non-hospital behavioral healthcare settings that are surveyed under the *CAMBHC,* such as residential treatment facilities and mental health centers, were worded exactly the same as the hospital standards. But now, as Chapter 5 discusses (see p. 87), while the restraint and seclusion standards in the *1999–2000 Comprehensive Accreditation Manual for Hospitals (CAMH)* are new, the standards in the *1999–2000 Comprehensive Accreditation Manual for Behavioral Health Care (CAMBHC)* have not changed. Therefore, the one-to-one correspondence between the standards in the two manuals no longer exists. Because the extent of the modifications to individual hospital standards is minor—aside from the new standards—however, this chapter's discussion of hospital standards is also generally applicable to the behavioral healthcare standards. (The restraint and seclusion standards in the *CAMBHC* are TX.3.1 through TX.3.1.3.3.)

In some acute care and general hospitals with psychiatric units, both sets of restraint and seclusion standards—the 21 standards applicable to behavioral healthcare settings in hospitals and the eight standards applicable to nonbehavioral health care—apply. Therefore, these hospitals will probably require two different sets of policies and two different staff training programs to comply with both sets of standards, even though there is considerable overlap in intent between the two.

What this chapter covers

This chapter presents information and advice for each individual restraint and seclusion standard in the *CAMH* that cover

- what the standard means,
- how surveyors score the standard,
- how surveyors evaluate the standard, and
- what an organization should do to comply with the standard and to demonstrate compliance to JCAHO surveyors.

This chapter concludes with a discussion of standards that directly impact the use of restraint and seclusion but are in sections of the *CAMH* other than the *Care of the Patient (TX)* chapter. (There are similar standards in the *1999 Comprehensive Accreditation Manual for Behavioral Health Care [CAMBHC]* and the *1999 Comprehensive Accreditation Manual for Ambulatory Care [CAMAC]*.)

Occasionally, the meaning and wording of what a JCAHO standard requires differ from what the same standard's scoring guidelines seem to require. We resolve this discrepancy by recommending ways to satisfy the requirements of standards, intent statements, and scoring guidelines together, thereby surpassing the JCAHO's minimum level of compliance. (Technically, an organization must comply with scoring-guideline requirements only, since those are what surveyors use to evaluate an organization's compliance.)

In addition, a few of the scoring guidelines in the software that is installed in the laptop computers that all surveyors now use to record and score survey findings appear to differ from the published scoring guidelines. This chapter indicates those instances of which we are aware.

And finally, some JCAHO standards result in higher frequencies of Type I Recommendations than others do. This chapter provides the percentages of healthcare organizations surveyed between January and December of 1998 that received Type I Recommendations on each standard. Organizations can use this information to set priorities for survey preparation because surveyor emphasis in the future might be the same as in the past.

The advice and suggestions in this chapter are one expert's opinion, and readers should not interpret them as the only means of satisfying JCAHO requirements or as the JCAHO's official statement.

Requirements beyond the JCAHO

When healthcare organizations decide which measures to implement to comply with the JCAHO standards, they must also remember to comply with the requirements of authorities other than the JCAHO. For example, many states and some local jurisdictions regulate restraint and seclusion use through laws or licensing regulations. An organization should follow whichever requirements are more stringent to ensure compliance with both the JCAHO and governmental authorities. In addition, because restraint and seclusion are high-risk procedures that are obvious targets for medical malpractice and liability lawsuits, an organization must develop its policies and practices to satisfy the recommendations of its own attorneys and liability insurance companies.

Standards regarding restraint use in behavioral healthcare settings

TX.7.1: Restraint or seclusion use within the organization is limited to those situations with adequate, appropriate clinical justification.

What it means

This standard is the parent standard that encompasses all other subsidiary standards relating to restraint and seclusion in hospital and ambulatory settings. If a hospital scores low on a subsidiary standard, that score might also impact its score on TX.7.1.

The key words in this standard are *adequate* and *appropriate clinical justification* for restraint or seclusion. The criteria for justification of restraint and seclusion should be written into an organization's

- medical staff bylaws, rules, regulations, and policies and procedures;
- administrative policies and procedures;
- nursing policies and procedures; and
- clinical practice guidelines and similar materials that are commonly referred to as *clinical parameters, clinical pathways, clinical algorithms,* and *protocols.*

Patient records should explain how a restraint or seclusion episode was justified (i.e., how the episode met clinical restraint or seclusion criteria). Furthermore, the documentation of the episode must be clearly in accordance with organizational policies and other procedures.

Note: The "Example of Implementation" feature in the CAMH *is a frequently used source of information regarding compliance with a particular JCAHO standard. The Example of Implementation for standard TX.7.1 is actually a carryover from the 1996 manual and does not correspond to the 1999 standard. The outdated example clearly deals with care for patients in a general hospital, while the 1999 TX.7.1 applies only to behavioral healthcare patients.*

How it is surveyed

Surveyors are likely to base the score of TX.7.1 on their overall impression of a hospital's practices that they've gathered through staff interviews, observations during tours, and even patient interviews. Review of documentation in patient records might also influence scoring of this standard, although TX.7.1 is not a standard that the JCAHO officially lists for systematic evaluation during the Closed Medical Record Review session.

How it is scored

Scoring of this standard is subjective, since surveyors must determine whether "adequate and appropriate justification" was present for restraint or seclusion use, according to hospital policies. A score of 1 indicates compliance; 3 (there is no score of 2), compliance "with a few minor exceptions"; and 5 (there is no score of 4), noncompliance.

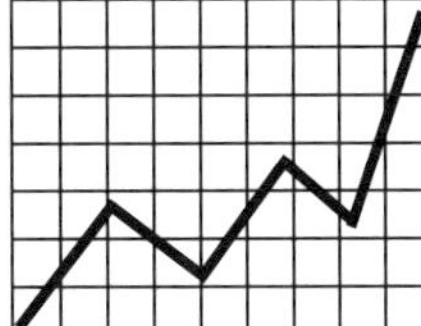

1.7% of hospitals received a score of 3, 4, or 5 on this standard in 1997; therefore, it is not a "problematic" standard (a standard is "problematic" if more than 5% of surveyed hospitals receive a 3, 4, or 5 on it).

What to do

Achieving a score of 1 on TX.7.1 requires compliance with all of its subsidiary standards. A hospital should therefore strive to comply with all the subsidiary standards, and TX.7.1 will take care of itself.

TX.7.1.1: Organization leaders support limited, justified use of restraint or seclusion through appropriate:

What it means

This standard serves as the stem or foundation for the next seven standards (TX.7.1.1.1 through TX.7.1.1.7) and is not scored. The key words in this standard *are limited, justified use of restraint*—words that emphasize the JCAHO's concern with reducing restraint and seclusion use and using restraint and seclusion only when absolutely necessary.

How it is surveyed

This standard is not surveyed, since it is not scored and surveyors do not need to determine a hospital's compliance with it.

How it is scored

TX.7.1.1 is not scored.

What to do

Since this standard is not scored, compliance with it depends upon compliance with its subsidiary standards, discussed below.

TX.7.1.1.1: Plans, policies, and priorities;

What it means

This standard is concerned with the organizational documents that describe and regulate an organization's use of restraint and seclusion—the plans, policies, and procedures—and the setting of priorities (presumably as specified in the organization's plans) to support appropriate use of restraint and seclusion.

How it is surveyed

Surveyors examine documents, such as the plan for professional services, patient care policies, and other relevant materials, in the document review session and can ask about them in any other survey sessions when the topic comes up. Surveyors are also likely to request additional information during the leadership and department directors' interviews—particularly if they find the documents insufficient when they first examine them—at which point organizational representatives can supplement whatever is in the documents.

How it is scored

TX.7.1.1.1 is scored at LD.1.1.1 (in the *Leadership (LD)* chapter of the *CAMH*), which covers the organization's plans. The scoring guidelines state that compliance with this LD standard depends upon how well an organization's plans, policies, and procedures address important care and hospital-wide functions. Because TX.7.1.1.1 specifically refers to LD.1.1.1, surveyors expect to see that a hospital deals with restraint and seclusion in its planning (i.e., restraint must be covered as part of planning).

The scoring guidelines for this standard do not require objective data and do not provide a framework that surveyors can use to score the standard. Therefore, surveyors have a significant measure of discretion in scoring it. Survey experience suggests that whenever leadership neglects a major planning issue, such as restraint planning, the organization will be scored as noncompliant even if it covers the majority of key issues in its planning. Scoring guidelines require surveyors to issue a score of 1, 3, or 5. But because the standard is "capped" at 3 in 1999—meaning the standard is limited in the extent to which it can be scored as noncompliant—failure to plan for restraint use and reduction will most likely result in a score of 3. Surveyors can still score it as a 4 or 5; the cap is applied in the official report.

Less than 1% of surveyed hospitals scored below 1 on this standard in 1998.

What to do

To comply with this standard, a hospital should ensure that its plans, policies, and procedures

- consider the allocation of resources for staffing, staff training, and the social aspects of the environment of care (see standard EC.4 in the *Management of the Environment of Care* chapter of the *CAMH* for more information on the social aspects of the environment of care);

- include specific discussion concerning the reduction or prevention of restraint and seclusion use; and

- comply with the new standards, since even those hospitals that have policies and procedures that fully comply with the old TX.7.1 might find that additions and revisions are needed.

TX.7.1.1.2: Human resource planning;

What it means

This standard applies to human resource (personnel) issues as they relate to restraint and seclusion—a new emphasis for most hospitals. In the past, restraint and seclusion use was considered a routine part of the staff's overall workload. But under this standard, a hospital's allocation of staff—as well as staff training and supervision—must account for the workload produced by applying restraint and seclusion in addition to the workload produced by searching for and using less restrictive alternatives.

Presumably, the JCAHO is emphasizing through this standard that excessive or improper use of restraint or seclusion can result from poor allocation of staff and inadequate training and that proper planning can reduce the need for personnel to deal with restraint and seclusion, since they are labor intensive to apply. This standard implies that healthcare organizations should prohibit use of restraint or seclusion to reduce the need for staff and that a high frequency of restraint or seclusion suggests inadequacy in staff training or the number of staff members (see Chapter 3, p. 60 for more discussion relevant to this issue).

How it is surveyed

Surveyors examine documentation demonstrating human resources planning, and they are likely to emphasize interviews with hospital leaders and department directors to assess compliance with this standard.

How it is scored

TX.7.1.1.2 is scored at standards LD.2.4 and LD.2.5 (in the *Leadership* chapter of the *CAMH*), which are concerned with the execution of department director responsibilities. To score LD.2.4, surveyors examine how well department directors use a sufficient number of qualified and competent staff, with the score based on the percentage of department directors who are in compliance. Surveyors score LD.2.5 by evaluating how well department directors determine the qualifications and competence of department staff who are not licensed independent practitioners (primarily nursing staff). The score for LD.2.5 is subjective, with 1 indicating compliance, 3 indicating that department directors are "not consistently" in compliance, and 5 signaling noncompliance. Survey experience reveals that surveyors do not emphasize either of these standards and only striking noncompliance will receive scores lower than 1.

Less than 1% of hospitals received a score of 3, 4, or 5 in 1998.

What to do

To comply with this standard, a hospital should

- make sure that its documents detailing the allocation of human resources—such as plans, staffing analyses, budgets, and workload estimates—take into account the necessary resources restraint and seclusion measures require;
- specifically mention restraint and seclusion in such human resources–related documents; and
- educate appropriate department heads and other hospital leaders on the measures taken to comply with this standard, so that those leaders can answer effectively when questioned during the survey.

TX.7.1.1.3: Staff orientation and education creating a culture emphasizing prevention and appropriate use and encouraging alternatives;

What it means

This standard requires that hospital culture—the informal and pervasive set of values, attitudes, and behaviors that dominate the work environment—emphasize the appropriate use of restraint and seclusion and use of alternatives. Many factors determine a hospital's culture, including the following:

- formal operating rules and policies;
- leadership directives and attitudes;
- characteristics by which new workers are selected, including personality, size, age, and gender;

- group process among workers;
- hospital tradition; and
- culture of the surrounding community.

Although the perception of a hospital's culture is considerably subjective, surveyors are likely to find evidence of the desired culture if a hospital's professional practice documents, training programs, and policy implementation emphasize restraint reduction (see "How it is surveyed" below).

How it is surveyed

To assess compliance with TX.7.1.1.3, surveyors

- determine the percentage of staff whose personnel records indicate restraint and seclusion orientation and inservice training;
- question frontline employees on what training the employees have had and what employees know about restraint and seclusion; and
- are likely to ask questions in the Leadership, Department Head, and Medical Staff Leadership interviews to assess the degree of emphasis on employee training and on creating a culture that promotes restraint reduction.

How it is scored

TX.7.1.1.3 is scored at HR.4 and HR.4.2 (in the *Human Resources* chapter of the *CAMH*). HR.4 requires orientation of recently hired staff, assessment of the abilities of recently hired staff, and training for staff who perform new duties. HR.4.2 requires hospitals to offer ongoing inservice training and education to improve staff competency.

Scoring of HR.4 is determined by the percentage of staff who complete orientation and the percentage of staff who participated in inservice training during the year before survey. Although standard TX.7.1.1.3 emphasizes the appropriate hospital culture, its scoring depends upon the presence of formal training programs. Although restraint and seclusion are only two of the many areas that must be covered in orientation and inservice training, surveyors will almost certainly evaluate restraint and seclusion orientation and inservice training.

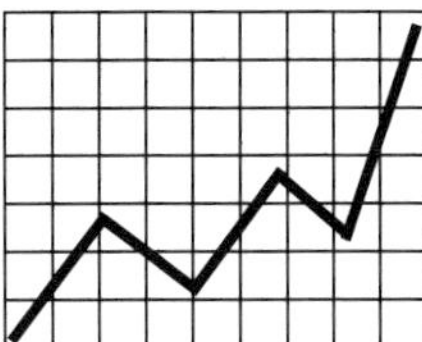

3.3% of surveyed hospitals received a score of 3, 4, or 5 on HR.4 in 1998, although there is no indication that noncompliance scores related to restraint or seclusion. Less than 1% of hospitals received a score of 3, 4, or 5 on HR.4.2.

What to do

Changing a hospital's culture is a difficult, uncertain process. Changes regarding the use of restraint and seclusion are most likely to result from a whole series of actions—including the response to the JCAHO's new standards. But, because the scoring of TX.7.1.1.3 relates specifically to staff orientation and inservice training, hospitals ideally should have measurable processes to demonstrate compliance with the standard.

To meet this standard, a hospital should

- make sure that orientation for newly hired staff and training for other staff who perform new duties includes specific, practical information about application of restraint and seclusion;

- measure staff members' absorption of orientation materials at the completion of orientation. For example, a hospital might administer a written exam that describes restraint scenarios and requires staff to propose alternatives to restraint, or it might require staff to actually demonstrate how they will apply restraints to patients; and

- include a review of restraint and seclusion—and emphasize the importance of using alternatives to restraint and seclusion—during periodic inservice training, which the JCAHO requires for a number of other areas as well.

TX.7.1.1.4: Patient and, when appropriate, family education;

What it means

This standard requires hospitals to provide education to patients and patients' families about reasons for and alternatives to restraint and seclusion. Educating patients' families can facilitate their assistance in reducing the need for restraint, or at least in minimizing the negative aspects of the experience for patients.

Education is essential when a patient—or a family member acting as a legal guardian—is asked to consent to restraint, since consent is valid only if the person granting it is aware of

- the reasons restraint is needed;
- the positive and negative aspects of restraint;
- the alternatives to restraint; and
- the consequences of refusing to consent.

Patient education should emphasize the reasons the patient might require restraint or seclusion and how the patient can avoid restraint or seclusion. An example that demonstrates appropriate patient education in a behavioral healthcare setting is a staff member's telling a patient: "You have been acting in a way that frightens the staff because they think you might be about to attack one of them. To avoid having anyone injured, we are going to have to put restraints on your arms and legs. As soon as you have calmed down and no longer seem to be about to attack, we will release you."

How it is surveyed

Surveyors assess patient and family education primarily through

- examination of documentation in patient records—usually checklists or progress notes—showing that patients (and families, when appropriate) receive education on key issues;

- interviews with patients and staff in which surveyors ask questions regarding the routine practice of educating patients and specific educational efforts for particular patients; and
- examination of policies and procedures that describe educational efforts (such policies and procedures should be available during the document review session, but surveyors might also request them in other survey sessions).

How it is scored

Standard TX.7.1.1.4 is scored at PF.4 and PF.4.2 (in the *Patient and Family Education [PF]* chapter of the *CAMH*). PF.4 requires hospitals to plan, support, and coordinate activities and resources that provide patient and family education. A score of 1 indicates appropriate planning, support, and coordination of educational activities and resources; 3, the hospital does not do so consistently; and 5, these activities are insufficient or not done.

PF.4.2 reiterates a frequent theme in JCAHO standards: the educational process must be multidisciplinary and collaborative. A score of 1 means the educational process is completely multidisciplinary and collaborative; 3 indicates inconsistent compliance; and 5, noncompliance.

Surveyors evaluate restraint and seclusion education as one part of the whole educational effort, so compliance with the requirements of these restraint and seclusion standards will not completely determine the scores for PF.4 and PF.4.2. However, failure to deal with restraint or seclusion educational issues might well lead to a score of 3 in either or both of the standards.

Less than 1% of surveyed hospitals received scores of 3, 4, or 5 on PF.4 and PF.4.2 in 1998.

What to do

To comply with TX.7.1.1.4, a hospital should

- make sure that all of its educational plans, protocols, and guidance for employees include restraint and seclusion;

- prepare educational materials on restraint and seclusion, and train employees how to use the materials with patients and families;

- incorporate restraint and seclusion education in any patient and family educational materials and in the forms that the hospital uses to document educational efforts;

- monitor the documentation of educational activities in medical records to check that evidence of required activities is present; and

- prepare department heads, other leaders, and patient care staff so that they can discuss the restraint and seclusion component of the hospital's patient and family education activities with JCAHO surveyors and others.

TX.7.1.1.5: Assessment processes that identify and, when appropriate, prevent potential behavioral risk factors;

What it means

This standard requires that staff assess restraint or seclusion use prior to its application in every instance—even in emergency use. There are two types of assessments: those done regularly as part of routine patient care and those performed as emergency procedures so that restraint or seclusion might be quickly applied. Much of what this standard requires is included in the routine assessments of patients who have serious physical or mental illness.

The key words in TX.7.1.1.5 are *identify* and *prevent*. Hospitals must assess risk factors that suggest an increased likelihood of the need for restraint or seclusion. Such factors might include a patient's

- diagnosis;

- current physical and mental status (including symptoms);

- treatment plan and course;
- personality (including the methods the patient uses to deal with physical and mental stress); and
- history (including previous episodes that led to use of restraint or seclusion as well as the methods that were effective in ending the need for restraint or seclusion).

For example, staff should evaluate a patient admitted with severe paranoid delusions and a history of violent outbursts to determine if, during the course of treatment, he or she might need and respond to restraint or seclusion. Staff members should analyze each risk factor to determine whether steps can be taken to reduce or eliminate that factor, thereby preventing the need for restraint. Questions staff should consider during their analysis are these:

- Can the patient tolerate the use of major tranquilizers?
- Is there a history of effective use of tranquilizers?
- In the past, have family members or therapeutic team members successfully modified the delusions or at least gotten the patient to not respond to them?

Emergency assessments are necessarily brief and should focus only on relevant issues. While staff must perform a restraint-use assessment and consider alternatives to restraint before actually using it, staff can place evidence of the assessment in a patient's medical record *after* the patient is restrained and the emergency is over.

How it is surveyed

To assess compliance with this standard, surveyors

- review policies relating to restraint and seclusion in the document review session;

- are likely to interview hospital and medical staff leaders—including department chairs—to ask about restraint and seclusion assessments;
- are likely to question nursing staff and to examine open medical records during the tour of patient care units to determine how well staff perform and document restraint and seclusion assessments; and
- examine several patient assessment reports that relate to restraint or seclusion during the closed medical record review session.

How it is scored

TX.7.1.1.5 is scored at PE.1.1, PE.3.1, PE.6, PE.7, and PE.8 (in the *Patient Assessment [PE]* chapter of the *CAMH*).

PE.1.1 requires hospitals to conduct "further assessments"—intensive examinations of relevant areas, issues, and problems—based on factors discovered during the initial assessment of patient's physical, psychological, and social condition. The percentage of patient records in compliance with this standard in the closed medical record review determines the score. Surveyors might, however, examine and count open medical records or base their scores on observations during tours and interviews.

PE.3.1 requires hospitals to base patient care on patient needs, priorities, and clinical information—rather than on issues that are unrelated to patient needs, such as staffing patterns or the facility's architectural design. Therefore, hospital staff must consider all available information for each patient to best identify and determine how to meet the patient's needs. Scoring of this standard is done exactly as it is for standard PE.1.1, described above.

PE.6 requires staff to consider the special assessment needs of patients who receive treatment for emotional or behavioral disorders. The intent statement for this standard requires hospitals to assess include a number of items in the assessment of such patients, such as the patient's history of mental, emotional, behavioral, and substance use problems or a psychosocial assessment. Although none of the items listed in the intent statement relates specifically to restraint or seclusion, many are relevant. For example, if, upon admission, a patient exhibits the same behavioral problem for which he or she was restrained in the past, staff should note this in the patient's written assessment as required by the item in the intent statement that says: "the history and treatment of behavioral problems." By including patient history in the assessment, hospital staff can review the precipitants of previous restraint episodes when considering how to avoid future ones. Scoring for PE.6 is done exactly as it is for PE.1.1, described above, except that PE.6 is capped at 4.

PE.7 applies primarily to patients who receive treatment for alcohol or chemical dependency. As with PE.6, the intent statement of this standard lists a number of items that staff must include in assessments of such patients. Scoring is done exactly as it is for PE.1.1, described above.

PE.8 is similar to PE.6 and PE.7, but is specific for patients who are abuse or neglect victims. Scoring is done exactly as it is for PE.1.1, described above.

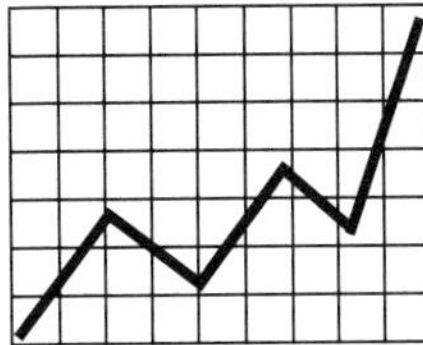

1.1% of surveyed hospitals received a score of 3, 4, or 5 on PE.7 in 1997. Less than 1% of hospitals received scores below 3 on standards PE.1.1, PE.3.1, PE.6, and PE.8.

What to do

To comply with TX.7.1.1.5, a hospital should

- make sure its policies and other documents pertaining to patient assessments, such as checklists and standardized forms, include restraint and seclusion provisions (one effective approach is to create a list that staff should consider for every patient placed in restraint or seclusion and incorporate that list in organizational policies and forms);

- orient staff on the use of patient assessment documents to prepare them for JCAHO survey;

- gather and review the medical records of patients who were placed in restraint or seclusion to check that appropriate assessments were performed and documented;

- be prepared to show that patient records contain all required items and that the items were completed either before or immediately following restraint or seclusion application; and

- consider developing a single form or template that contains space for every required JCAHO item, space for physician orders, progress notes, nursing notes, and a nursing observation flow sheet that can be used for every episode of restraint or seclusion.

TX.7.1.1.6: Design and delivery of patient care; and

What it means

This standard provides criteria for issues related to an effective patient care process as it pertains to restraint and seclusion, including the following:

- Patient care plans must take into account patients whose symptoms, diagnoses, or status indicate high risk for restraint or seclusion.

- Care plans should indicate that staff first try less restrictive alternatives to restraint or seclusion and also specify the circumstances under which restraint or seclusion will be used.

How it is surveyed

During their tour of patient care settings, surveyors assess a hospital's process for creating and documenting individual patient care plans as they relate to restraint and seclusion by

- interviewing staff;

- examining open medical records;

- possibly interviewing patients; and

- evaluating clinical settings.

How it is scored

TX.7.1.1.6 is scored at TX.1 and TX.1.1. TX.1 requires that hospitals individualize every patient care plan. Surveyors score TX.1 based on the percentage of patients whose care is individualized and appropriate, as reflected in the review of closed medical records.

TX.1.1 requires that settings for the provision of treatment services are appropriate to patient needs. Regarding restraint and seclusion, this standard requires that hospitals make the appropriate settings available to either help avoid the need for restraint or seclusion, or to ensure that restraint or seclusion is safe, effective, humane, and brief. Surveyors score TX.1.1 based on the percentage of patients for whom settings and services are appropriate, as reflected in the review of closed medical records. However, surveyors are free to use open medical record evaluations or tour experiences and interviews in their scores.

As with many of the standards discussed in this chapter, restraint and seclusion are only two of a large number of issues surveyors consider when scoring TX.1 and TX.1.1.

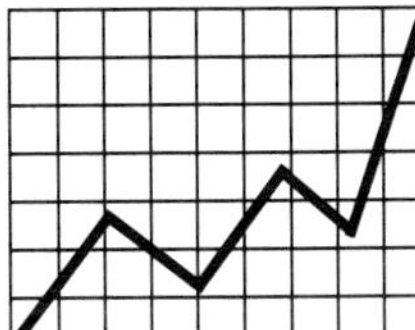

2.9% of surveyed hospitals received scores of 3, 4, or 5 in, although there is no indication that the scores were linked specifically to restraint or seclusion. Less than 1% of hospitals surveyed in 1997 received a score of 3, 4, or 5 on TX.1.1.

What to do

A hospital should make sure that

- every patient care plan addresses whether the patient might need restraint or seclusion;
- when staff unexpectedly place a patient in restraint or seclusion, they reevaluate and appropriately modify the care plan both to reduce the likelihood of further need for restraint or seclusion and to ensure that any future episodes are in accordance with the plan; and

- staff evaluate patient care settings to assess their effectiveness in reducing the need for restraint and seclusion and the appropriateness of administering restraint and seclusion in them. (Such assessments should include staffing patterns and the social milieu, in addition to physical characteristics.)

TX.7.1.1.7: The development and promotion of preventive strategies and use of safe and effective alternatives.

What it means

This standard emphasizes preventing restraint and seclusion and using alternatives to them. It is slightly different from TX.7.1.1.3, which concerns organizational culture and staff orientation and training. Hospitals can demonstrate compliance with TX.7.1.1.7 by having policies and procedures that require, and staff training programs on, the use of preventive measures and alternatives before restraint or seclusion application.

Some examples of preventive or alternative measures for treating patients at high risk for restraint or seclusion include

- high levels of staff observation and interaction with patients;

- encouraging family members to visit patients frequently and for long periods of time; and

- using mechanical devices and physical environments that control dangerous behaviors without physically restricting patients.

(Chapter 4 discusses other alternatives to restraint and seclusion.)

How it is surveyed

Surveyors will subjectively estimate compliance with this standard through

- review of documents—primarily policies and plans—in the document review session;

- various leadership interviews; and
- observations and interactions during the hospital tour.

How it is scored

Surveyors score TX.7.1.1.7 by evaluating the use of preventive and alternative strategies. A score of 1 represents compliance; 2, compliance with a few minor exceptions; 3, inconsistent compliance; 4, rare compliance; and 5, noncompliance. Indications of satisfactory compliance are left to each surveyor to determine. Scoring guidelines for this standard are vague and rely on surveyor discretion.

Less than 1% of surveyed hospitals received scores of 3, 4, or 5 on this standard in 1997 and 1998.

What to do

A hospital should develop a list of preventive and alternative strategies for treating patients at high risk for restraint or seclusion and determine what resources are necessary for executing each strategy, such as

- staff training;
- alternative devices;
- architectural changes; or
- changes in existing policies.

After assembling its list of preventive and alternative strategies, a hospital should

- first focus on the strategies that it can implement in a short period of time;
- prepare long-term plans for executing the strategies that require resources that are more difficult or time consuming to obtain;
- immediately train staff to implement the less complicated strategies; and

- make sure hospital leaders are familiar with the implementation process for the less complicated strategies and with implementation plans for the other, more labor-intensive strategies.

TX.7.1.2: Performance-improvement processes identify opportunities, when appropriate, to reduce restraint or seclusion use.

What it means

This standard requires hospitals to use their performance improvement (PI) systems to reduce the use of restraint and seclusion. The intent statement for this standard makes it clear that the JCAHO considers restraint and seclusion to be high-risk and problem-prone treatments. Therefore, the JCAHO expects healthcare organizations to collect data about restraint and seclusion and make the reduction of these treatments a high priority. (Organizations that believe that their use of restraint and seclusion is so infrequent that reduction is not a priority should be prepared to prove this.)

In addition, the intent statement for TX.7.1.2 requires that hospitals make it a top priority to study the reasons for multiple episodes of restraint and seclusion on single patients and also study the frequency of restraint and seclusion use by staff type. The latter requirement allows hospitals to determine whether particular staff characteristics lead to a greater likelihood of incidents that precipitate the use of restraint or seclusion. For example, studies might reveal that night-shift nursing staff are more inclined to restrain patients who tend to wander, or female staff members are more inclined to restrain adolescent male patients. If any such correlation is found, subsequent investigations should center on eliminating their causes and finding preventive measures. (Note that the intent statement for this standard recognizes that although, in principle, physician orders should initiate most episodes of restraint, the reality is that front-line staff in minute-to-minute contact with the patients usually initiate restraint and then rely on the physician to ratify the decision.)

How it is surveyed

During leadership interviews, surveyors are likely to ask about a hospital's inclusion of restraint and seclusion in its performance improvement program. In addition, surveyors assess PI efforts regarding restraint and seclusion in at least one of the three activities devoted specifically to performance improvement: the PI overview, the PI coordinating group interview, and the PI team interview. Surveyors also expect that restraint-related performance improvement activities meet the requirements outlined in the *Performance Improvement* chapter of the *CAMH*: when there is an adverse event or unexpected, significant statistical deviation, organizations must collect quantitative data and then statistically analyze and intensively evaluate it (essentially a root-cause analysis).

How it is scored

TX.7.1.2 is scored on its own (not, as might be expected, at standards in the *Performance Improvement* chapter of the *CAMH*). A score of 1 represents compliance; 2, compliance with minor exceptions; 3, inconsistent compliance; 4, rare compliance; and 5, noncompliance.

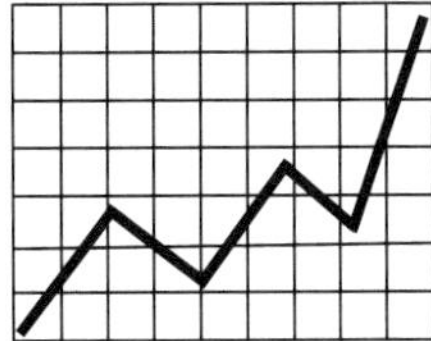

This standard was one of the top 40 most problematic standards in 1997: 6.4% of surveyed hospitals received a score of 3 or worse. In the first half of 1998, over 7% of hospitals received a score of 3, 4, or 5.

What to do

Since the basic thrust of the new JCAHO standards is to reduce the frequency of restraint and seclusion use, a wise course of action for an organization is to assume that whatever its frequency of restraint and seclusion use, it can further reduce it. To achieve this reduction, a hospital should

- systematically collect data about the frequency of restraint and seclusion use, including the characteristics of patients and settings where restraint and seclusion occur;
- identify causative elements that lead to episodes of restraint or seclusion (what the intent statement of TX.7.1.2 terms *root causes*);
- evaluate each root cause in relation to cost or ease of modification to develop an effective plan to reduce the frequency of restraint and seclusion; and

- employ benchmarking methods—comparisons with similar hospitals whose restraint and seclusion policy is effective and outstanding, or comparisons with published reports about appropriate rates of restraint and seclusion use—to evaluate its own use of restraint and seclusion.

The JCAHO now requires (by the intent statement of PI.3.1.1) that hospitals treat restraint and seclusion as one of the specific measures for regular measurement and assessment (similar to the review of operative and other procedures and the review of medication use). Including restraint and seclusion in PI efforts is not optional.

TX.7.1.3: When restraint or seclusion is used, organization policy and procedures guide appropriate and safe use.

What it means

This standard requires hospitals to have policy and procedure statements that deal with appropriate and safe use of restraint and seclusion—not just techniques for applying restraint and seclusion. While the JCAHO has traditionally required medical staff approval of such policies and procedures, the intent statement of TX.7.1.3 simply states that "appropriate staff" must approve these policies and procedures, thereby allowing other groups to carry out the review and approval in organizations that do not have medical staffs. In a hospital, medical staff still have the responsibility unless there is some good reason for another group to have it.

The intent statement lists nine elements that policy and procedure statements must include to ensure the protection of patient rights, dignity, and well-being. These nine elements essentially repeat the requirements of the other standards relating to restraint and seclusion and are excerpted here:

The organization

- protects and preserves the patient's rights, dignity, and well-being during restraint use;
- bases use on the patient's assessed needs;
- makes decisions about least restrictive methods;

- assures safe application and removal by competent staff;
- monitors and reassesses the patient during use;
- meets patient needs during use;
- limits individual orders to licensed independent practitioners;
- time-limits orders; and
- documents in the medical record when restraint or seclusion is used.

TX.7.1.3 pertains to the existence of policy and procedure statements and the approval of these statements by the appropriate authority—not with policy and procedure execution.

How it is surveyed

Surveyors emphasize restraint and seclusion during documentation review and the tour of the patient care units. Hospitals should have a set of the policies, procedures, protocols, and training materials relating to restraint and seclusion available for the document review session. During tours, surveyors are likely to question employees about their knowledge of policies and procedures and to evaluate employees' use of policies and procedures if they encounter a patient in restraint or seclusion during the tour. (Strictly speaking, however, surveyors should not score noncompliance at this standard if they witness staff not following policy.)

How it is scored

TX.7.1.3 is unique because it is the only restraint and seclusion standard scored in the *Care of the Patient (TX)* chapter of the *CAMH* that is capped. It is capped at 3.

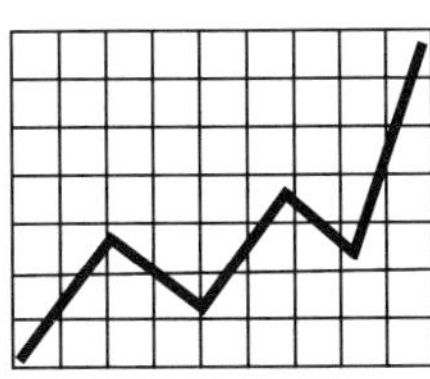

This standard was one of the top 40 most problematic standards in 1997. 3.5% of surveyed hospitals received scores of 3, 4, or 5 on it. (Although TX.7.1.3 is capped, surveyors can still score it as a 4 or 5; the cap is applied in the official report.) This standard was not among the top 40 most problematic, however, during the first half of 1998.

Scoring guidelines for this standard are clear for a score of 1: the required policy and procedure statement is present, complete, and approved by the appropriate staff. Scoring for the other levels of compliance, however, is complex:

- A score of 2: The hospital's policy and procedure statement adequately considers the nine required elements "with a few minor exceptions." (The interpretation of "minor" depends on the surveyor's judgment.)

- The guidelines are even more complex for a score of 3: The organization's policy does "not consistently" address the required elements (again involving surveyor judgment), and policy approval by appropriate staff is 95% to 99% (but it is not made clear how to measure the extent of policy and procedure approval).

- A score of 4: The policy "rarely" deals with the required elements.

- A score of 5: The hospital does not have the required policy and procedure, and approval is less than 95%.

One possible explanation for this puzzling set of scoring guidelines is that it was written incorrectly. In any case, it is difficult to determine the meaning of a percentage of policy approval.

What to do

The key action for a hospital to take is to develop or revise its restraint and seclusion policy and procedure statements to make sure they address the nine essential elements the intent statement lists. It is probably most effective for a hospital to develop a single set of policies and procedures that meets all the new requirements, since a number of other standards also require the development or revision of policies and procedures.

To comply with TX.7.1.3, a hospital should

- clearly separate and organize its policy and procedure statement and any other key documents relating to restraint. The JCAHO does not require that these be separate documents, but having the restraint documents together in one place rather than lost among a collection of other documents will simplify the surveyor's review;

- provide documentation showing "appropriate staff" (in a hospital, this is most likely the medical staff) approval of policies and procedures. Hospitals should place this documentation directly in the policy and procedure statement itself—although other options are available, such as recording statements in committee minutes;

- be sure that policies and procedures cover all situations that might be considered restraint or seclusion;

- clearly explain how it determined what "appropriate staff" means (in most cases, this is the medical staff, which does not require further explanation); and

- make sure leaders are generally familiar with the contents of the policy and procedure statement and can discuss how policies and procedures are approved.

TX.7.1.3.1 (formerly TX.7.1.3.2): Individual orders for restraint or seclusion are consistent with organization policy.

What it means

This standard requires restraint and seclusion orders by licensed independent practitioners to be consistent with hospital policy. TX.7.1.3.1 is the parent standard for a number of more detailed standards covering orders for restraint or seclusion.

How it is surveyed

Since TX.7.1.3.1 is not scored, surveyors will not review it separately. They will, however, include it in the survey of its subsidiary standards, so a hospital's compliance level with TX.7.1.3.1 will affect the scores of other standards.

How it is scored

The JCAHO does not discuss the practical meaning of this standard in the scoring guidelines because it isn't scored.

What to do

To comply with this standard, a hospital should

- make sure its restraint and seclusion policies cover issues relating to restraint and seclusion episodes that licensed independent practitioner orders initiate;
- check that policies specifically state such orders must comply with all other relevant standards;
- educate and train appropriate staff, such as licensed independent practitioners (mostly physicians), to know the policy requirements and limits that govern the nature and execution of their orders;
- train and educate personnel (primarily nurses) who carry out such orders—including how personnel should handle situations in which they determine that an order is not acceptable under the policies; and
- consider using printed forms, rubber stamps, or reminder stickers in the records of patients who are restrained or secluded to guide physicians and nurses in meeting all requirements.

TX.7.1.3.1.1 (formerly TX.7.1.3.2.1): Patient rights, dignity, and well-being are protected during restraint or seclusion use.

What it means

TX.7.1.3.1.1 echoes several standards previously discussed in this chapter. It requires organizations to protect the rights, dignity, and well-being of patients who are restrained or secluded via an order.

A hospital must consider four specific items, listed in the intent statement of TX.7.1.3.1.1, regarding patients who are restrained or secluded:

- respect for the patient as an individual;
- safety and cleanliness of the restraint or seclusion environment;
- assurance that patients are still able to receive and participate in care; and
- protection of patients' modesty, visibility, and body temperature.

How it is surveyed

Surveyors assess compliance with TX.7.1.3.1.1 by

- examining policies;
- interviewing hospital leaders, staff, and sometimes patients;
- observing activities during the hospital tour; and
- reviewing the open medical records of patients who are or have been in restraint or seclusion.

How it is scored

Scoring for this standard occurs at standard RI.1 (in the *Patient Rights and Organization Ethics* chapter of the *CAMH*), which addresses ethical issues in providing care. RI.1 scoring is determined by how completely organizations address the nine specific items listed in its intent statement and by the percentage of staff who can explain how they "support and protect patient rights."

Scoring for RI.1 is as follows:

- 1 indicates that a hospital addresses all of the listed items and that 91% to 100% of interviewed staff can explain the hospital's ethical approach to the surveyor's satisfaction;

- 2 is given if a hospital omits one of the nine listed items or if 90% to 99% of interviewed staff can explain the hospital's ethical approach to the surveyor's satisfaction;

- 3 indicates noncompliance with two or more of the nine listed items, or 75% to 90% of interviewed staff can explain the hospital's ethical approach to the surveyor's satisfaction;

- 4, 50% to 74% of staff can explain the hospital's ethical approach to the surveyor's satisfaction; and

- 5, less than 50% of interviewed staff can explain the hospital's ethical approach to the surveyor's satisfaction, or the hospital has no method to address ethical issues.

Restraint and seclusion are only two of a large number of issues surveyors consider when scoring this standard. Less than 1% of hospitals surveyed in 1997 and 1998 received a score of 3, 4, or 5.

What to do

To comply with this standard, an organization should

- develop a policy that protects patients' rights, dignity, and well-being during application of restraint and seclusion;

- develop a corresponding procedure statement that describes in detail how the policy is executed;

- include the policy and procedure statements in staff orientation and inservice educational programs and consider providing them (or a summary) in educational materials regarding restraint and seclusion given to patients and their families (see TX.7.1.1.4);

- document its efforts to comply with this standard. For example, a hospital could include documentation—such as a checklist that shows regular review of the physical environment—in the records of restrained or secluded patients;

- document any specific issues—such as a special effort made to facilitate a patient's continued participation in treatment during restraint and seclusion—in patient records; and

- heavily emphasize this issue to staff during last-minute survey preparation, since scoring guidelines focus heavily on quantifying results of staff interviews. Organizations might consider providing staff with "cheat sheets" (e.g., reminder pocket cards) to assist staff in answering questions.

TX.7.1.3.1.2 (formerly TX.7.1.3.2.2): Restraint or seclusion use is based on the assessed needs of the patient.

What it means

This standard requires hospitals to assess patients appropriately before applying restraint or seclusion via an order, either as part of routine initial assessments or through emergency assessments.

Hospital policy should state that qualified staff perform such assessments. Each assessment should take into account the patient's clinical condition and treatment plan in relation to restraint and seclusion.

Hospitals should address four items listed in the intent statement of TX.7.1.3.1.2:

- The training and qualifications of individuals authorized to direct emergency application of restraint or seclusion in the absence of licensed independent practitioners (usually registered nurses)

- The licensed independent practitioner's responsibility for emergency restraint use or use without an order or through an order

- A review of repeated use or prolonged use of restraint and seclusion with a single patient

- The organizational policy on restraint and seclusion

The intent statement specifically points out that a hospital cannot base a decision to apply restraint or seclusion solely on a patient's history. Nor can a hospital apply restraint or seclusion for punishment or staff convenience. Rather, it must depend on a patient's immediate needs and interactions with others. The documentation of assessments in the patient's record serves as required clinical justification for restraint or seclusion. In other words, the patient's record should show that staff considered the possible use of restraint or seclusion in the initial assessment or that emergency use was based on an appropriate, if hurried, assessment at the time of application. Follow-up orders (and preferably the progress note as well) from the physician or other licensed independent practitioner involved should ratify emergency restraint use. Furthermore, only individuals who are specifically authorized by hospital policy and have had the training that hospital policy specifies should direct emergency restraint application.

How it is surveyed

Surveyors evaluate compliance with this standard by

- scrutinizing policies;

- interviewing hospital leaders, staff, and patients; and

- examining patient records.

How it is scored

Scoring of TX.7.1.3.1.2 is based on whether uses of restraint or seclusion are responsive to assessed patient needs. A score of 1 indicates compliance; 2, compliance with a few minor exceptions; 3, compliance is not consistent; 4, rare compliance; and 5, noncompliance.

What to do

To comply with this standard, a hospital

- should develop guidelines for assessing patients before using restraint and seclusion;
- should incorporate these guidelines into the restraint and seclusion policy statement;
- should develop a training program (or training criteria) for individuals authorized to direct emergency use of restraint or seclusion;
- will probably need to create separate, more detailed guidelines for nursing staff to follow when they must do emergency evaluations in the absence of licensed independent practitioners; and
- should check that staff members document every use of restraint or seclusion in the patient's record, which should include details of the patient assessment and the clinical justification for restraint or seclusion.

TX.7.1.3.1.3 (formerly TX.7.1.3.2.3): The least-restrictive safe and effective restraint or seclusion method is employed.

What it means

This standard requires organizations to use the least restrictive methods of restraint or seclusion that are safe and effective for patients. Restraint use ranges from least restrictive—tying a cotton glove on a patient's hand while the arm is left free—to very restrictive—tying four limbs and waist to a bed. There are far fewer variations of seclusion, but they can range from use of a patient's own room to use of a special room with all furnishings removed and special clothing for the patient. When alternative methods are available, a hospital should have a policy specifying how it selects methods for restraint or seclusion.

The intent statement of TX.7.1.3.1.3 says the determination of which method to use depends on

- policy;
- staff experience with the patient;
- assessment and monitoring of the patient; and
- patient and staff safety.

How it is surveyed

To assess compliance with TX.7.1.3.1.3, surveyors

- examine a hospital's restraint and seclusion policies;
- interview hospital leaders, staff, and patients; and
- examine patient records.

How it is scored

Scoring for this standard is similar to the other standards in this group, although it is perhaps somewhat more subjective because surveyors must determine, with their own judgement, whether the least restrictive, safe, and effective restraint and seclusion methods are used. A score of 1 indicates compliance; 2, compliance with minor exceptions; 3, inconsistent compliance; 4, rare compliance; and 5, noncompliance.

What to do

To comply with TX.7.1.3.1.3, a hospital should

- make sure that its restraint and seclusion policy describes its various methods and resources for applying restraint and seclusion—including what space, equipment, and trained staff are available;
- rank its restraint and seclusion methods in terms of restrictiveness;
- educate physicians and those authorized to direct emergency restraint or seclusion to order the least restrictive method available;

- describe in its policy specific behaviors that trigger application of restraint or seclusion and make sure the policy states that the final decision is at the discretion of the senior clinician on the spot;

- orient and regularly retrain staff in how to select restraint and seclusion options;

- consider developing a checklist to assist staff in selecting the most appropriate restraint and seclusion methods; and

- make sure staff document the restraint and seclusion process in the patient's record for every restraint or seclusion episode.

TX.7.1.3.1.4 (formerly TX.7.1.3.2.4): Restraint or seclusion is used correctly by competent, trained staff.

What it means

This standard requires organizations to determine what a competent, trained staff member is and then make sure that those staff members are the only ones who apply restraint devices and initiate or terminate seclusion.

The intent of TX.7.1.3.1.4 also requires the involvement of competent staff in two phases of the restraint and seclusion process: initiation or application and removal or termination. Presumably, these processes involve different skills.

In sharp contrast to standards in prior years, TX.7.1.3.1.4 requires organizations to ensure that each staff member who initiates or terminates restraint is competent and trained. In the past, most organizations operated under the assumption that all members of the nursing staff could be allowed to initiate restraint in emergency situations in the absence of physicians. Sometimes this authority was limited to a group designated in terms of their administrative positions, rather than their specific training. In addition, many organizations permitted any nurse to release patients from restraint or seclusion. This current standard, however, requires organizations to train employees who apply and remove restraint or seclusion. Therefore, the organization should also periodically evaluate restraint and seclusion skills.

How it is surveyed

To assess compliance with TX.7.1.3.1.4, surveyors

- examine hospital policy on staff training and competency evaluation;
- interview hospital leaders and staff; and
- examine the personnel files of individuals authorized to apply and remove restraint and seclusion.

How it is scored

Scoring for this standard is done at standard HR.5, which requires hospitals to perform periodic competency assessments of employees using accurate job descriptions. Scoring of HR.5 is not capped and is based on the percentage of staff members' records that indicate competency assessments were completed. Failure to comply with the restraint and seclusion aspect of HR.5 alone will not necessarily lead to a significant scoring problem, because dealing with restraint and seclusion is almost always just one small part of an employee's responsibilities. However, even if a personnel record lacks just one competency assessment, the record is considered noncompliant, although commonly surveyors use their discretion.

What to do

To comply with TX.7.1.3.1.4, an organization should

- state in its restraint and seclusion policy the competency requirements staff must meet to be able to authorize emergency restraint. The policy should also specify the requirements staff must meet to be able to apply or remove restraint devices or to carry out seclusion;
- conduct evaluations and offer appropriate training programs to assist staff in meeting the requirements;
- be sure to record completion of competency requirements in each authorized staff member's personnel record;

- develop a list of personnel who have achieved the competency designation so that this information is readily available to assist in personnel assignments; and

- educate hospital leaders and supervisors in competency requirements and policy so that they can describe the system to surveyors.

TX.7.1.3.1.5 (Formerly 7.1.3.2.5): Patients in restraint or seclusion are monitored and reassessed appropriately.

What it means

This standard requires hospitals to monitor and reassess patients in restraint and seclusion to the extent described in their policies. However, policies must require monitoring at least every 15 minutes, and reassessment at least at the expiration of every time-limited order before a hospital can extend or renew the order. Adequate documentation of monitoring and reassessment is critically important.

Monitoring can be accomplished in several ways:

- observation of the patient through a window or peep-hole in a door;

- observation by means of closed-circuit TV; and

- observation during a visit to the patient when vital signs are checked.

Reassessment is almost always completed by an in-room observation of the patient, including a brief physical and mental examination. (Note that renewal of the order by a licensed independent practitioner must be based on a face-to-face assessment. Reassessment should focus on whether there is a continued need for restraint or seclusion, as well as on the patient's general physical and mental condition.)

How it is surveyed

To assess compliance with this standard, surveyors

- review the hospital's restraint and seclusion policy;

- interview hospital leaders and staff;
- examine the medical records of patients who have been in restraint or seclusion; and
- might observe the treatment of any patients in restraint or seclusion during the hospital tour.

How it is scored

The subjective evaluation of the extent and appropriateness of the monitoring of patients who are in restraint and seclusion determines the score of this standard. A score of 1 indicates compliance; 2, compliance with minor exceptions; 3, inconsistent compliance; 4, rare compliance; and 5, noncompliance.

2.5% of surveyed hospitals received a score of 3, 4, or 5 on this standard in 1997.

What to do

To comply with TX.7.1.3.1.5, a hospital should check that its restraint and seclusion policy

- establishes the minimum frequency of monitoring patients—at least every 15 minutes;
- designates exactly which items staff observe during monitoring;
- outlines the changes in a patient's condition that trigger consideration of release from restraint or seclusion and/or consultation with a physician;
- states which categories of personnel are authorized to monitor patients; and
- specifies how often patients are reassessed during restraint or seclusion (at least at each renewal or extension of an order), who does reassessments, and how they are done.

In addition, a hospital should consider using a medical record form (usually called a nursing observation flow sheet) to facilitate observation recording.

TX.7.1.3.1.6: Patient needs are met during restraint or seclusion use.

What it means

This standard requires hospitals to meet the major needs of patients during restraint and seclusion. Such needs include food, liquids, access to the toilet, exercise, circulatory well-being, and protection of skin integrity. This standard is consistent with, but not quite the same as, the one above it (TX.7.1.3.1.5). As previously noted in the discussion of TX.7.1.3.1.5, the frequency with which patient needs are observed and documented is dependent on policy but must be at least every 15 minutes. An organization usually pays attention to patient needs in conjunction with monitoring and reassessment, but monitoring might be more frequent than just when patient needs are fulfilled. For example, some hospitals require constant, continuous observation and documentation of those observations every 15 minutes, but they allow access to the toilet and fluids once an hour.

Consider attending to patient needs in the following ways:

- attend to needs that require the most frequent attention—liquids, circulatory well-being, and toilet access—at least hourly;
- attend to food needs three times a day;
- attend to exercise and skin integrity needs three times a day, but not at mealtimes;
- offer bathing at least once every 24 hours for prolonged episodes of restraint and seclusion; and
- pay attention to patients' emotional needs and protection of their dignity and respect. (A hospital must define and specify what these items mean and how to monitor them.)

How it is surveyed

To assess compliance, surveyors

- examine a hospital's restraint and seclusion policies;
- ask questions regarding the restraint and seclusion policies and their execution during leadership and staff interviews;
- review the records of patients in restraint or seclusion during the hospital tour and check whether attention to patient needs is appropriately documented; and
- review patient records during the closed medical record review session.

How it is scored

The surveyor's subjective interpretation of evidence regarding the fulfillment of patient needs determines the score. A score of 1 represents total compliance; 2, a few minor exceptions; 3, inconsistent compliance; 4, rare compliance; and 5, noncompliance.

What to do

To comply with TX.7.1.3.1.6, a hospital should

- make sure its restraint and seclusion policy specifies how the hospital attends to patient needs;
- educate hospital leaders and staff regarding the policy and its execution; and
- determine how it will document attention to patient needs. (As with TX.7.1.3.1.5, a hospital should consider implementing a medical record form devoted to restraint and seclusion to facilitate consistent documentation.)

TX.7.1.3.1.7 (Formerly TX.7.1.3.2.7): Restraint or seclusion use is ordered by a licensed independent practitioner.

What it means

This standard emphasizes the point made in a number of other standards: that only licensed independent practitioners can give orders for restraint or seclusion—almost always a physician in this context. The JCAHO expects healthcare organizations to explicitly state this requirement in hospital policy. In hospitals that recognize professionals other than physicians as licensed independent practitioners, hospitals must consider whether they will extend authority to order restraint and seclusion to nonphysicians. (In some states, laws or regulations prohibit this.)

Specifically, a hospital's policy must specify

- which individuals may give restraint and seclusion orders (in other words, some hospitals might further limit restraint and seclusion authority only to certain licensed, independent practitioners);

- which individuals may receive orders when they are verbal or given via telephone (usually registered nurses);

- which professionals who are not licensed independent practitioners have the authority to directly use restraint and seclusion in emergencies in the absence of a licensed independent practitioner; and

- the time interval in which a licensed independent practitioner must issue a regular order following emergency use of restraint or seclusion (the intent statement for the standard requires the interval to be one hour or less).

Aside from the JCAHO requirements, many states also regulate other aspects of restraint and seclusion. Therefore, healthcare organizations must consider local requirements when developing their restraint and seclusion policies.

How it is surveyed

To assess compliance, surveyors review the relevant policy during the document review session, and they might interview hospital leaders and staff. The scoring guidelines, however, make it clear that surveyors will emphasize the open and closed medical records examination when scoring this standard.

Compliance with TX.7.1.3.1.7 should be heavily emphasized since it is one of the most problematic JCAHO standards. Common reasons for noncompliance with this standard include the discovery of one or more records that document episodes in which restraint or seclusion was initiated without an order or in which restraint or seclusion continued beyond the expiration of a valid order without a new order.

How it is scored

Scoring of TX.7.1.3.1.7 is based on the documentation of orders initiating or continuing episodes of restraint and seclusion. A score of 1 indicates 100% of restraint and seclusion episodes are initiated by proper orders; 2 indicates 95% to 99%; 3, 90% to 94%; 4, 80% to 89%; and 5, less than 80%. Note that scoring counts episodes and not records (i.e., a record might include more than one episode, each of which is counted separately).

12% of surveyed hospitals received a score of 3, 4, or 5 on this standard in 1997.

What to do

To comply with this standard, a hospital should

- be sure that its restraint and seclusion policy covers the standard requirements relating to orders for restraint and seclusion, including which individuals are authorized to issue orders and under what circumstances, who might receive verbal and telephone orders, who might initiate emergency procedures, etc. Hospital policy should also address the general responsibilities of licensed independent practitioners;

- educate hospital leaders and staff, including all licensed independent practitioners, regarding the policy and its execution; and

- periodically review the medical records of patients who experienced restraint and seclusion to be sure that records demonstrate that the policy was followed.

TX.7.1.3.1.8 (formerly TX.7.1.3.2.8): Orders for restraint or seclusion use define specific time limits.

What it means

This standard and its intent statement outline the following specifications for restraint and seclusion orders:

- Each order must specifically state the maximum duration of restraint (i.e., "up to four hours"). According to the standard, the maximum permissible time limit is four hours for adults, two hours for patients aged 9 to 17, and one hour for patients under age 9. Hospital policy and state law can also limit the length of time. But regardless of any predetermined limits, the JCAHO still expects each individual order to specify the maximum length of time a patient can be restrained before he or she is released or reassessed.

- The hospital's restraint and seclusion policy, protocols, or documents must contain criteria that guide a staff member's decision to exercise the option of releasing a patient from restraint or seclusion before the expiration of an order.

- If a patient exhibits the same problematic behavior after release from restraint or seclusion (but before the order expired) as he or she did prior to restraint application, then staff can place the patient back in restraint or seclusion without an additional order for the period of time remaining on the original order. If the patient exhibits problematic behavior during the release period that is different from the behavior that initiated the original order, however, staff must obtain a new order for restraint or seclusion.

- A "licensed, qualified, and authorized individual" can reassess and renew an order for a period of time up to the maximums stated above (four hours, two hours, or one hour, as appropriate) *provided the initial order authorizes it*. This individual might renew an order repeatedly, up to a total of 24 hours, at which time a licensed independent practitioner must perform the face-to-face reassessment and write a new order. (This extension of the order might not be permissible in some states.)

- A licensed independent practitioner or a licensed, qualified, and authorized individual must perform reassessments on a face-to-face basis to determine if there is a continued need for restraint or seclusion. When a licensed independent practitioner writes an order to initiate restraint or seclusion that does not provide for a continuation or extension of the order, the licensed independent practitioner must perform a face-to-face assessment before writing a new order (i.e., the new order cannot be a telephone order based on a nurse's description of the need for a new order). For example, if an order was written for four hours of restraint and did not authorize continuation of it, then a doctor must come after four hours to see the patient if nurses believe that there is a continued need for restraint.

How it is surveyed
To assess compliance with TX.7.1.3.1.8, surveyors

- examine a hospital's restraint and seclusion policy during the document review session;

- are likely to discuss the policy and its application during interviews with hospital leaders and staff;

- are likely to examine the records of patients who are in restraint and seclusion during the hospital tour;

- are likely to question staff regarding records; and

- heavily weigh observations from the closed medical record review session—the most important scoring element of this standard.

TX.7.1.3.8 is perennially one of the most problematic standards, primarily because physicians fail to write restraint or seclusion orders that meet JCAHO requirements or the policies of their hospitals. Specifically, physicians neglect to make the restraint or seclusion order time-limited, or to specify a limit that is within the maximum time the standard allows.

How it is scored

The percentage of restraint and seclusion orders that indicate time limits determines the score for this standard. A score of 1 indicates 100%; 2, 95% to 99%; 3, 90% to 94%; 4, 80% to 89%; and 5, less than 80%.

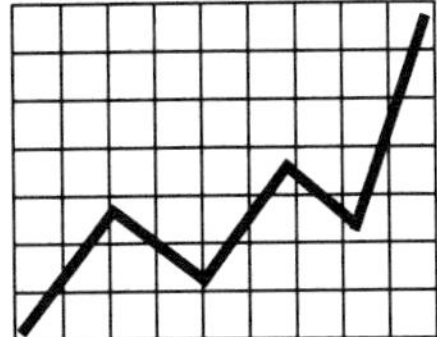

TX.7.1.3.1.8 was the most problematic standard in 1997. 37.9% of surveyed hospitals received scores of 3, 4, or 5. In the first six months of 1998, 10.5% did.

What to do

To comply with TX.7.1.3.1.8, a hospital should

- be sure that its restraint and seclusion policy deals with each of the issues this standard covers;
- be sure that hospital leaders and staff are familiar with the restraint and seclusion policy;
- as part of ongoing medical record review, review the records of patients who were restrained or secluded to assess whether the records reflect compliance with all aspects of this standard;
- develop criteria for training and competency assessments to determine who is a licensed, qualified, and authorized individual and can therefore continue restraint and seclusion orders for up to a maximum of 24 hours;
- develop a list of staff members who meet the above criteria; and
- establish a set of guidelines for authorized staff to make decisions regarding continuation of restraint and seclusion orders.

TX.7.1.3.2 (Formerly TX.7.1.3.3): Documentation in medical records reflects organization policy.

What it means

This standard requires that reports of every episode of restraint and seclusion include

- justification;
- an order that meets hospital policy (and JCAHO standards);
- a description of efforts to protect the patient's rights and fulfill the patient's physical and psychological needs; and
- regular monitoring of the patient.

How it is surveyed

To assess compliance with TX.7.1.3.3, surveyors supervise a review of medical records during the survey. To do this, staff compare records against a JCAHO form, which lists all of the standard-based requirements for records. The results of the comparisons are tallied and yield the score for each of the standards listed on the form.

Surveyors also evaluate a small number of open records during their tours of patient care units. The results from these examinations are added to those from the closed medical record reviews to produce the final score.

This standard (or its predecessor) has been perennially among the top problematic standards. Common reasons for noncompliance include failure to document justification for use of restraint or seclusion in records; failure to adequately document attention to patient needs (this is probably best recorded in a flow chart or similar form); and use of an order that does not comply with JCAHO standards or hospital policy.

How it is scored

The percentage of restraint or seclusion episodes in the evaluated medical records that meet the JCAHO and hospital policy requirements determines the score for this standard. A score of 1 indicates that 100% of records were in compliance; 2, 95% to 99%; 3, 90% to 94%; 4, 80% to 89%; and 5, less than 80%.

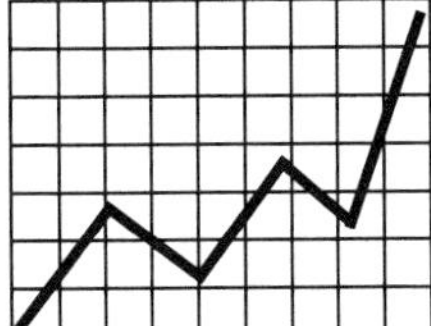

This standard was among the top 40 problematic standards in 1997. 15.2% of surveyed hospitals received scores of 3, 4, or 5. 4.7% of surveyed hospitals did during the first six months of 1998.

What to do

To comply with TX.7.1.3.2, a hospital should

- in each periodic review of medical records, review a representative sample of records that document restraint or seclusion episodes; and
- be sure that record entries for restraint or seclusion episodes include
  - clinical justification for the use of restraint or seclusion;
  - a valid, time-limited order from a licensed independent practitioner or adequate justification for use in an emergency; and
  - evidence that staff monitored and paid attention to patient needs during the restraint or seclusion episode, in accordance with JCAHO standards and hospital policy.

Standards regarding restraint use in medical and surgical settings

TX.7.5: The organization's leaders determine the organization's approach to the use of restraint in the care of nonpsychiatric patients, which limits its use to those situations where there is appropriate clinical justification.

What it means

TX.7.5 is the parent standard that encompasses several other subsidiary standards (TX.7.5.1, TX.7.5.2, TX.7.5.3, TX.7.5.3.1, TX.7.5.3.2, TX.7.5.4, TX.7.5.5). Noncompliance with any of these subsidiary standards can negatively impact the scoring of TX.7.5. This standard particularly emphasizes leadership's role in finding an approach to reducing restraint use.

How it is surveyed

The principal means of evaluating compliance with this standard is discussions during the leadership interview and leadership responses to questions about restraint during the survey in general.

How it is scored

Scoring is basically subjective and focuses on the answer to two questions:

- Are episodes of restraint use clinically justified?
- Have organization leaders taken the lead in shaping a satisfactory approach to restraint use?

If the answer to both questions is "yes," the hospital receives a score of 1. According to published scoring guidelines, scores of 2 or 3 are awarded when leadership's influence is obvious but clinical justification is lacking for a few restraint episodes. Scores of 4 or 5 mean that restraint is not clinically justified much or most of the time.

In practice, scoring depends on compliance with each question independently. For example, if clinical justification is found for every episode but the organization's leadership has not been involved in developing policies for restraint use, the organization can receive a score of 5.

What to do

To comply with this standard, a hospital should

- focus on complying with subsidiary standards (listed above), since success on this standard depends on full compliance with every standard that falls under it;
- ensure that leadership participates in restraint policy development and supervises the execution of the policy;
- in preparation for the survey, remind the leadership group of activities that

they carried out, and have them practice presenting this information as they would to surveyors;

- if statistics were collected regarding use of restraint (as they should have been), be sure leaders are aware of these statistics and what they mean (if statistics indicate unsatisfactory progress toward reducing use of restraint, leaders should be prepared to explain this to surveyors and describe the steps that are planned or are already being taken to bring about improvement).

TX.7.5.1: Performance-improvement processes seek to identify opportunities to reduce the risks associated with restraint use through the introduction of preventive strategies, innovative alternatives, and process improvements.

What it means

This standard requires restraint use to be part of the performance improvement program. Organizations must continuously collect, measure, assess, and, when indicated, improve all processes that are part of its PI program. The history of JCAHO's approach to restraint and the implication of standard TX.7.5 strongly imply that improvement, at least in part, equals a reduction in restraint use.

This standard is a revision of the 1996 standard, TX.7.1.2. If a hospital was in compliance with TX.7.1.2, it should have no difficulty with TX.7.5.1, even though the wording of TX.7.5.1 and its intent statement are somewhat different.

How it is surveyed

TX.7.1.2 is surveyed during several of the interview sessions. A common question surveyors ask in the leadership interview is "What is the hospital doing to reduce and improve the use of restraint?" Additionally, the same question is asked in the performance improvement coordinating group interview and the medical staff leadership interview. Some hospitals also schedule a presentation on performance improvement in restraint use as one of the performance improvement team presentations, or mention the team's efforts during the performance improvement overview. This type of presentation usually covers the issue without the surveyors' having to ask questions. Storyboards or other exhibits of performance improvement activities are good ways to showcase restraint-related PI activities.

How it is scored

Scoring is subjective and depends on the surveyors' impression of the effectiveness of the hospital's restraint-related performance improvement activities. Scoring guidelines mention scores of 1, 3, and 5, but surveyors might issue scores of 2 or 4 when appropriate. The guidelines also state that if restraint use is rare to the degree that organizations cannot obtain data, surveyors should give a score of 1.

What to do

To comply with TX.7.1.2, a hospital should

- incorporate restraint use into the hospital's performance improvement system and expect surveyors to scrutinize it;
- not treat restraint use as an optional PI area, even if the episode frequency is low;
- assign responsibility for monitoring and reducing restraint use to a specific group, similar to the groups that deal with medication use or the review of operative procedures;
- take action—and then immediately document that action—whenever the trend in restraint use is unfavorable or when an adverse event occurs; and
- prepare documents that show the trend in restraint use and report the analyses of the trend.

TX.7.5.2: Organization policy(ies) and procedure(s) guide appropriate and safe use of restraint.

What it means

This standard is a revision of the 1996 standard, TX.7.1.1.1, which concerns plans, policies, and priorities.

TX.7.5.2 requires hospitals to have a detailed document that describes the many aspects of its restraint reduction approach. Although the standard calls this document a "policy and procedure," JCAHO surveyors do not care what the document is titled—or even that all of the required elements are in a single document—as long as one or more documents contain all of the required elements.

The intent statement for the standard lists eleven "essential elements" that should be covered in the document and divides the elements into two groups (Group A elements are weighted slightly less by surveyors than Group B elements are, as explained under "How it is scored," below). Most of the elements clearly reflect good clinical practice and are required by other standards as well. The hospital's policy should describe or define each of the elements and the means by which the hospital attains and monitors the element.

The Group A essential elements that should be considered in the policy are the following:

- protection of the patient's safety, rights, dignity, and well-being;
- restraint is need-based, as demonstrated in the patient's assessment;
- utilization of the most effective, but least restrictive, method of restraint;
- restraints are safely applied and removed by staff trained to use the particular method or device;
- qualified staff monitor the patient during restraint; and
- patient needs are met during restraint (e.g., for liquids, nourishment, toilet access, movement and exercise, skin integrity, and psychological well-being).

The Group B essential elements that should be considered in the policy are the following:

- how staff deal with any unique risks or problems of patients who are in "vulnerable" populations, such as "emergency, pediatric, and cognitively or physically limited" groups;

- patient and family education efforts regarding restraint;

- only licensed independent practitioners order restraint;

- any renewal of orders for restraint are in accordance with state law; and

- all episodes of restraint are documented in individual patient records.

The medical staff (or equivalent) and nursing leadership (it is up to the hospital to define this term) should approve the document or documents that contain these essential items. In most hospitals, the administration will also approve the document.

This standard and its intent statement essentially lay out most of the structure around which a restraint program should be built, in contrast to the 1996 approach, in which many issues were each covered by a single standard (which is still the case for the 1999 behavioral healthcare standards).

How it is surveyed

Compliance with this standard is carefully reviewed during the Document Review Session, when the hospital's policy is examined. In principle, the surveyors check to see that the policy considers each of the required elements. In practice, however, surveyors never have enough time to examine each of the documents available during the document review, and they usually scan quickly those that they do review. But since restraint is currently a high-priority issue, it is likely that at least one of the surveyors will devote time to read the policy carefully and thoroughly.

Surveyors look for indications of how the policy is implemented. They ask to see open medical records of patients who were restrained, interview staff about restraint practices, and they might talk with patients and family members about restraint. Any indications that staff do not follow policy requirements or are not educated about them might result in a lower score on this standard or might be counted against one of the other standards.

How it is scored

Scoring for this standard is both subjective and relies heavily on surveyor judgment. Surveyors ask two questions to score this standard:

- Are all the required elements present in the policy?

- Have the medical staff, nursing leadership, and other appropriate groups approved the policy?

According to the published guidelines, if the answer to both questions is "yes," the organization receives a score of 1. Organizations receive a score of 2 if one Group B element is absent but the approvals are present; a score of 3 if one Group A element or two or three Group B elements are absent or if approvals are "not consistently" obtained; a score of 4 if four of five elements (presumably from either group) are missing; and a score of 5 if more than five elements are missing or if there are none of the requisite approvals.

Because the scoring is subjective and because the absence of a required item is difficult to establish to the satisfaction of all concerned, it can lead to controversy. For example, "protection of patient rights" can appear in any of several documents a hospital develops, and even when not explicitly stated, such protection is often implied. Therefore, when surveyors determine that the element that deals with patient rights is lacking, they might not be able to convince hospital representatives of that "fact."

Another facet of this standard that can confuse scoring is what should happen, for instance, when the policy covers the protection of patient rights and dignity but not patient well-being—the third of the three elements required to be protected. The guidelines do not explain what should happen in terms of scoring in this scenario.

What to do

To comply with TX.7.5.2, a hospital should

- develop a policy that covers all the required elements and do so in a practical, meaningful manner;
- determine which elements require specific training for certain staff members (such as nursing staff who apply and remove restraint devices) and add a description of that training to the policy;
- obtain the necessary approvals for the policy;
- develop documents that go along with the policy (e.g., special forms that can be used for doctor's orders, progress notes, or for recording attention to patient needs).
- train staff on the policy as a whole, as well as the elements of the policy that require specific training for specific groups;
- prepare reminders for front-line staff on the key issues and actions of the policy so that they can easily comply with the standards and can impress surveyors with their familiarity with the policy; and
- give equal emphasis to Group A and Group B elements. (Although the JCAHO differentiates the importance of the two groups slightly, it generally considers both to be equally important.)

TX.7.5.3: Any use of restraint (to which these standards apply) is initiated pursuant to either an individual order (standard TX.7.5.3.1) or an approved protocol (standard TX.7.5.3.2).

What it means

This standard is an introductory statement for the two standards that follow it (TX.7.5.3.1 and TX.7.5.3.2). It is not scored, and compliance depends upon compliance with both of its subsidiary standards. The standard does not make clear what surveyors should do with restraint episodes that were not ordered or were not a part of a protocol, even though the wording of the standard suggests such episodes should be scored here (such episodes will probably be scored as non-compliant at standards TX.7.5 or TX.7.5.2).

How it is surveyed

This standard is not individually surveyed.

How it is scored

This standard is not scored.

What to do

See the discussion for standards TX.7.5.3.1 and TX.7.5.3.2.

TX.7.5.3.1: Individual orders for initiation and renewal of restraint are consistent with organization policy(ies) and procedure(s), and are consistent with the patient's needs and clinical condition.

What it means

The intent of this standard represents a significant change from that of its predecessor, 1996 standard TX.7.1.3.2. The 1999 standard itself is a straightforward statement of what preceding standards require. Nonetheless, the details of the intent statement require careful examination.

The intent statement says that in a situation in which restraint is clinically justified (the statement omits the word "emergency," which was used in the 1996 standard) but a licensed independent practitioner is "not available to issue such an order," a registered nurse may initiate restraint application without an order for up to 12 hours. In contrast, 1996 standard TX.7.1.3.2 stated that "an individual" (therefore not necessarily a nurse) could be authorized (by hospital policy) to apply restraint, but only in an emergency. Furthermore, for medical/surgical patients in 1996, there was no defined time limit for the use of emergency restraint and no requirement that a licensed independent practitioner be notified.

However, almost all hospitals in 1996 that permitted emergency restraint without an order were more restrictive than the standard, and they required that a licensed independent practitioner be notified immediately, who would provide an order within one hour (which is still required in behavioral healthcare settings). By means of the intent statement of the 1999 standard, the JCAHO has invited hospitals to considerably increase nurses' authority.

This increased authority allows nurses to restrain an individual if necessary, even in a nonemergency situation. A licensed independent practitioner (presumably the patient's physician) does not need to be informed for 12 hours, at which time the physician can give a verbal or telephone order without seeing the patient. The physician does not have to see and examine until 24 hours has elapsed (with one exception: When a change in a patient's condition is the basis for applying restraint, a licensed independent practitioner must be notified immediately. Presumably however, the nurse can still apply restraint to deal with an emergency until the licensed independent practitioner can respond). It is not clear whether a nurse who initiates restraint without an order and then terminates it before the 12 hours have elapsed is required at any time to notify a licensed independent practitioner. Regardless, good clinical practice indicates that as soon as is practicable the patient's physician should be notified, even if restraint has been discontinued.

Some hospitals might choose to invest nurses with this new additional restraint authority, while others might choose not to or might be prohibited from doing so by state laws or regulations. Most likely, however, this change in the JCAHO standard will start a movement in the direction of allowing nurse discretion regarding the use of restraint. Hospitals that elect to use this new authority are advised to restrict its use to designated registered nurses, not just any registered nurse, and to require designated nurses to complete additional training and to undergo competency testing.

Hospital policy should govern when orders for restraint are appropriate, what must be done as part of an assessment, what the documentation should consist of, etc. The intent statement for the standard specifies that renewal of the order after 24 hours must be done by a licensed independent practitioner and be based on an examination.

The intent statement also includes a new provision: A deviation from policy regarding monitoring of the patient or release from restraint before expiration of the order is permissible if the order allows for the deviation. The purpose of this provision is not explained. Hospitals are advised not to take advantage of the opportunity to permit less frequent monitoring of restrained patients, since doing so increases the risk of injury to the patient and consequent liability if something goes wrong.

How it is surveyed

The main determinant for scoring this standard is the closed medical record review. However, surveyors also examine the restraint policy, interview staff members about the execution of the policy, examine open records of patients who have been restrained or who are in restraint, and possibly interview patients and their families.

How it is scored

Published scoring guidelines for this standard involve subjective judgment because a score of 2 requires compliance "with a few minor exceptions"; 3, "not consistently" compliant; 4, "rarely" compliant; and 5, never compliant. The guidelines make it clear that surveyors should evaluate individual orders (i.e., documentation in the medical records) and that the order must include the name of the author (who must be a licensed independent practitioner), timeliness (both in relation to when the restraint episode occurred and the requirements stated in policy), and content (as required by the policy). The guidelines are not specific regarding the evaluation of situations in which a nurse applied restraint pending an order. Surveyors will almost certainly use the hospital's policy as the basis of evaluation of such episodes.

What to do

To comply with TX.7.5.3.1, a hospital should

- write a policy that meets all JCAHO and state requirements;

- consider taking advantage of the new power given to nurses to initiate restraint (if state laws or regulations permit) and if so, include this in the policy with instructions to guide the designated nurses (instructions should include the nature of the assessment nurses should complete and how to document the findings); and

- determine which nurses are designated (usually by position, rather than by name) and the content of the training program for those nurses, then train those nurses and document their competency evaluations.

TX.7.5.3.2: Protocols for restraint use contain criteria to ensure only clinically justified use.

What it means

This standard replaces the four 1996 standards that dealt with restraint protocols (TX.7.1.3.1, TX.7.1.3.1.1, TX.7.1.3.1.2, and TX.7.1.3.1.3). The 1996 standards broke new ground because they permitted "qualified staff members" (usually registered nurses) to use protocols as the basis for initiating restraint and for keeping a patient restrained for an indefinite period without an order from a licensed independent practitioner. Although this approach was permissible in some states, many hospitals were reluctant to utilize the authority and believed the JCAHO did not provide clear guidance on how to do so. The intent statement for the 1999 standard is much clearer in explaining what the Joint Commission means.

The 1999 intent statement explicitly requires that the restraint protocol

- be specific to surgical or medical conditions in which patient responses or behavior can inadvertently endanger the patient or interfere with the treatment (for instance, a protocol for the care of ventilator-dependent patients, which includes restraint as one element, is acceptable, whereas a general restraint protocol for a variety of diagnoses is not);

- contain a number of items: the nature and extent of the patient assessment and the criteria from that assessment—or other factors—that trigger the implementation of the protocol, a description of patient-monitoring requirements, the nature and frequency of reassessment, and the criteria for release from restraint;

- state that "authorized staff" can initiate restraint by following the protocol without an order from a licensed independent practitioner, and that restraint can be continued without an order as long as the criteria in the protocol are met;

- be subsidiary to—and within the requirements of—the hospital's restraint policy; and

- be approved by the medical staff (or equivalent), nursing leadership, and any other appropriate group (in most hospitals, the administration).

What the intent statement does not make clear are the following important questions:

- *Can restraint via protocol be continued indefinitely without any type of physician assessment or review?* We recommend that, at minimum, a physician assessment be required after 48 uninterrupted restraint hours. The assessment documentation should include the need for continued restraint use.

- *What are the requirements for inclusion as "authorized staff" (i.e., those who can initiate the protocol)?* We recommend that the requirements for "authorized staff" include:

  - a registered nurse in a supervisory position;
  - completion of a hospital-designed training program that covers protocol use and the initiation and termination of restraint, assessment, and patient/family education; and
  - periodic retraining and competency assessments.

- *Can a protocol be acceptable if it focuses on a particular symptom requiring restraint—such as wandering, or repeatedly removing lines or tubes—rather than on a diagnosis or procedure?* Our answer is "no." Based on what the JCAHO has stated, troublesome symptoms require a doctor's order.

- *Do* standardized procedures—*a term used in California to describe documents approved by multidisciplinary hospital committees and authorizing certain practices by nurses—meet the requirements for a protocol?* We suggest that they do.

- *How does the authority nurses have to use protocols mesh with—or differ from—the authority granted by standard TX.7.5.3.1 to initiate restraint for up to 12 hours without an order?* TX.7.5.3.1 seems to allow nurses a considerable amount of flexibility to initiate restraint, but it also limits the time for which the authority extends. Protocols do not seem to have time limits, although good clinical practice would require limits.

How it is surveyed

Surveyors consider this standard from two perspectives: (1) they examine the restraint policy, protocols that can trigger restraint, and evidence of the proper approval of the protocols during the document review session; and (2) they look for proper documentation of restraint in patient records for those who have undergone restraint. If any patients are in restraint during the survey, surveyors will review their records and evaluate how staff handle them. They will probably also interview staff to determine the staff's knowledge of policy and protocol. Closed medical records documenting restraint episodes are reviewed in the closed medical record session.

How it is scored

Scoring depends upon compliance in three areas: content of the protocol; approval of the protocol; and use of the protocol.

A score of 1 means requirements in all three areas are met. A score of 2 means that the content of the protocols lacks a few minor items or that application of the protocols complies with the protocols with a few minor exceptions. A score of 3 is given when either of the latter two issues lacks more than minor items or when the necessary approval of the protocols is incomplete. A score of 4 means that protocols or their application rarely meet requirements; and 5 is given when there is an absence of compliance in any of the three areas.

One of the predecessors of this standard, 1996 standard TX.7.1.3.1.2, generated scores of 3, 4, or 5 in 1.6% of surveyed hospitals in 1997.

What to do

To comply with TX.7.5.3.2, a hospital should

- decide whether to use the provision allowing protocols (if the hospital decides to do so, it should investigate what its state permits in this regard [this information will probably be in the state's nursing practice act or in the law or regulation on hospital licensure]);

- decide which diagnoses or procedures will be covered by protocols that include restraint;

- develop (or adapt from other facilities) the desired protocols;

- design the training and competency testing for "authorized individuals" and incorporate it into the policy on restraint;

- submit the protocols and the training/competency test to the appropriate bodies in the hospital for their review and approval, and, upon approval, incorporate these into the policy on restraint;

- develop any forms or documentation templates that will be used to facilitate the proper use of the protocol—and documentation of its use;

- train staff in their roles in authorizing, applying, monitoring, and releasing restraint; test staff competence; and periodically retrain and retest them.

TX.7.5.4: Patients in restraint are monitored.

What it means

This standard requires organizations to carefully observe restrained patients and to immediately respond to restrained patients' needs to prevent the damaging effects of restraint. Organizations typically monitor restrained patients through indirect observation by means of telemetry or closed-circuit TV; direct (face-to-face) observation; and during reassessment (involving measurement of vital signs, hands-on evaluation, and verbal interaction).

Hospital policy should describe the nature and extent of requisite monitoring, which must be done at least every two hours, as the standard's intent statement requires it to be (this is a new requirement). The requirement that hospitals include a detailed list of items that caregivers should observe as part of patient monitoring is another new element in the intent statement. This list of items should include patient well-being (both physical and mental); maintenance of patient rights, dignity, and safety; the possible switch to a less-restrictive alternative; indications for restraint removal; and appropriateness of restraint.

The intent statement does not define these terms, however, so hospitals should assume that they have a common-sense meaning. The intent statement also fails to mention the items most commonly considered during monitoring, perhaps considering these to be part of patient well-being. These items include the need for liquids, food, and exercise; evidence of skin irritation or breakdown; the need to use the toilet; washing; and bathing. Caregivers should document these items individually. It is a good idea for hospitals to develop a special form to facilitate patient monitoring and to make sure that patient monitoring is thorough and documented appropriately.

Note: This standard applies equally both to patients restrained by licensed independent practitioner order and those restrained by protocol.

How it is surveyed

The most important means of surveying this standard is the examination of closed medical records for documentation that shows proper monitoring. Surveyors also look at the policy on monitoring; interview staff about patient monitoring requirements, how staff monitor patients, and whether staff have discovered any adverse events during monitoring and, if so, how they dealt with the events; and possibly interview patients who were restrained and their families.

How it is scored

Scoring is subjective. Surveyors use the following criteria to score this standard:

- Is monitoring done in accordance with the standard and its intent?
- Is monitoring done in accordance with the hospital's policy?

If the answer to both questions is "yes," the score is 1. If it is "yes" with a few minor exceptions, 2; if the answer is "not consistently," the score is 3; if rarely, 4; and if no, 5. There is no guidance on how to score this two-part question if the answer to one part is consistently "yes," for example, and is "rarely" for the second part. This situation is different from the way similar standards that have more structured guidance are scored, and it is not clear if this difference is intentional.

The JCAHO requires surveyors to look separately at a number of specific items in evaluating compliance with this standard. Monitoring must comply with all of the hospital's requirements, as well as those of outside agencies that have jurisdiction. Monitoring should

- take place every two hours;
- include an evaluation of both physical and mental well-being and the protection of patient rights, dignity, and safety;
- consider if a less restrictive measure can be used;
- evaluate if circumstances have changed, which could lead to termination of restraint;
- consider whether restraint has been appropriately applied, removed, or reapplied; and
- be done only by qualified staff.

What to do

To comply with standard TX.7.5.4, hospitals should

- fully develop the portion of the restraint policy that outlines the requirements for monitoring;
- consider using special forms to document orders and descriptions of restraint monitoring;

- train staff in how to monitor patients and how to document monitoring (this training should emphasize that monitoring and assessment are multi-faceted activities that must be thoroughly documented);

- establish a review mechanism for documentation of restraint monitoring (which will likely be part of ongoing monitoring of medical records) and a means of responding immediately to unsatisfactory instances of monitoring.

TX.7.5.5: Each episode of restraint use is documented in the patient's medical record, consistent with organization policy(ies) and procedure(s).

What it means

This standard is similar to the 1996 standard, TX.7.1.3.3, and the 1999 standard, TX.7.1.3.2. TX.7.5.5 requires documentation of "each episode of restraint use," while the others deal with documentation in general and do not specify that individual episodes must be documented, although the standard has always been scored that way. The reason for the small difference in wording between this standard and the other two is not clear.

This standard provides the means for surveyors to evaluate overall restraint use rather than documentation alone. The standard requires organizations to have and to carry out a restraint policy that complies with JCAHO standards. The intent statement for this standard makes it clear that the policy on restraint must specify how documentation should be done, particularly in regard to frequency, format, and content. Content of the restraint documentation must include justification for restraint use (i.e., the less restrictive alternatives that failed); the patient's assessment; the order or protocol that initiated the episode; the monitoring protocol; documentation of attention to patient needs; the reassessment (if done); and the decision to terminate restraint.

How it is surveyed

Surveyors usually evaluate compliance with this standard during both the open and closed medical record reviews. Surveyors also informally evaluate how restraint is handled, however, during the survey. If they believe that restraint is not being applied in compliance with the standards, they will likely scrutinize medical records to substantiate their belief. If surveyors are in doubt about staff findings in the closed medical record review, a hospital should expect them to review the restraint records themselves and, if appropriate, to alter the score for this standard.

How it is scored

As mentioned above, scoring of this standard is based on a simple calculation of the percentage of examined medical records that comply with this standard. If 90 to 100% of the restraint episodes in the records comply, the score is 1; 80% to 89%, 2; 50% to 79%, 3; 25% to 49%, 4; less than 25%, 5. Although scoring guidelines describe the percentages as reflections of the medical records that are in compliance, surveyors have been instructed in the past to count individual documented episodes of restraint rather than entire records. This means that a record that reports three episodes of restraint, one of which is not compliant, will be scored as 66% compliant (i.e., 2 out of 3). This is different from the way other standards are scored in the medical record review.

Another aspect of the percentage-based scoring guidelines that make the scoring of this standard unique is that the percentages are less stringent in relation to the numerical scores than for a number of other standards whose scores are based primarily on medical record reviews. For example, IM.7.3.2.1, which requires an operative report that is dated and authenticated by the surgeon, requires 100% compliance for a score of 1 and gives a score of 5 for less than 50% compliance. On the other hand, standard TX.7.1.3.2, which is analogous to IM.7.3.2.1 but is applicable to behavioral healthcare settings, requires 100% compliance for a score of 1 and results in a score of 5 for anything less than 80% compliance.

Even though the percentage requirements for TX.7.5.5 are less stringent than for other standards, however, hospitals should not be tempted to be less concerned with this standard. It is still difficult to get a score of 1 because of the small sample size of examined records. Even in a large hospital, a relatively small number of records will be examined during the closed medical record review: perhaps 30 in the very largest hospital, and 15 to 20 in an average hospital. Out of that number, surveyors might ask for four or five restraint records that together, experience suggests, are likely to contain seven episodes of restraint. This means that if one record has one episode that is not compliant, it is mathematically impossible to get a score of 1. Two noncompliant episodes will lead to a score of 3 and a Type I Recommendation. Furthermore, while surveyors may increase the overall number of records reviewed—and thus reduce the impact of one noncompliant episode—by including open records that contain documentation of restraint episodes, they do not always do so, and such records are not always available.

What to do

To comply with standard TX.7.5.5, a hospital should

- be sure that the restraint policy, as well as the information management policy, discusses documentation of restraint episodes and lists the forms and information required in every record that reports a restraint episode;
- instruct all nursing staff on the essential requirements of restraint documentation and on the importance of their questioning orders that are not compliant with policy;
- include a regular review of restraint documentation in ongoing medical record reviews; and
- consider implementing concurrent record review for every report of restraint use. This means that as soon as a restraint episode occurs—preferably while it is still going on—a record reviewer (such as a member of the utilization management staff) checks to see that all required documentation is present. Any absent items should be immediately called to the attention of the responsible person for completion or correction.

Restraint-related standards in other chapters in the *CAMH*

PI.3.1.1: The organization collects data to monitor the performance of processes that involve risks or might result in sentinel events.

What it means

This standard requires facilities to collect data (which usually means collecting quantitative information, rather than merely case studies) about clinical activities and processes considered to be high-risk. Data collection should include measures of frequency in relation to such obvious variables as patient age, gender, diagnosis, precipitating event, time of day, alternatives to restraint that proved ineffective, etc.

The intent statement specifically lists restraint and seclusion as "an appropriate" standard to measure. The qualifying term "appropriate" certainly excuses a hospital that does not use restraint or seclusion from measuring it. A hospital that uses restraint could also presumably justify not studying restraint use—in accordance with the nonprescriptive tradition of the current standards—but it would have to make a strong case to satisfy surveyors that it was not appropriate to study it and to attempt to improve restraint use.

How it is surveyed

Surveyors may ask to see data and data analyses in any of a number of scheduled events during the survey, including the performance improvement overview and the leadership, medical staff, nursing leadership, patient care, and performance improvement coordinating group interviews. Surveyors might ask the personnel who present the data for interpretations of the data and for descriptions of any actions taken as a result of the findings.

How it is scored

Restraint is only one of the processes listed in the intent statement of this standard as appropriate to measure. Therefore, failure to measure restraint or seclusion will not necessarily result in noncompliance, provided that the hospital measures other appropriate processes. But failure to properly measure restraint or seclusion—or any other one of the listed processes—will likely lead to a score of no better than 2. To achieve a score of 1 requires having a plan or policy that specifies what will be measured and how often, and then consistently measuring performance in all high-risk areas—particularly the processes mentioned in the intent statement (which includes restraint and seclusion).

What to do

If an organization uses restraint or seclusion, then it must carry out the following actions to comply with standard PI.3.1.1:

- determine which aspects of restraint and seclusion it will measure and incorporate them into its performance improvement plan (the selection should consider the measures that have the most potential for improvement);

- develop an economical and effective measurement system (in doing so, the organization should consider what type of data collection forms are necessary and how it will collect and analyze the information from the forms);

- collect and analyze data—using statistical quality control techniques—for at least a year before the survey;

- implement performance-improvement strategies as indicated by the data analysis and then follow up on these actions to determine whether the improvement steps are effective; and

- document the entire process in such a way that is clear to surveyors (the organization should consider using graphic displays and storyboards, particularly if the improvement strategies were effective).

Other standards directly affected by compliance with restraint standards

The scoring of some standards that are in various chapters of the *CAMH* depends, in part, on compliance with restraint and seclusion standards. They include:

- LD.1.1.1, based on compliance with TX.7.1.1;

- LD.2.4 and LD.2.5, based on compliance with TX.7.1.1.2;

- HR.4 and HR.4.2, based on compliance with TX.7.1.1.3;

- PF.4 and PF.4.2, based on compliance with TX.7.1.1.4;

- PE.1.1, PE.3.1, PE.6, PE.7, and PE.8, based on compliance with TX.7.1.1.5;

- TX.1 and TX.1.1, based on compliance with TX.7.1.1.6;

- RI.1, based on compliance with TX.7.1.3.1.1; and

- HR.5, based on compliance with TX.7.1.3.1.4.

Chapter Seven

Creating Effective Plans, Policies, and Procedures

Policies, procedures, and other guidelines

Every organization that uses restraint must specify in great detail, in any of several different types of documents, a number of aspects regarding how it uses restraint. The JCAHO's 1996 standards regarding restraint and seclusion increased considerably the requirements for specific documents, and the 1999 revisions have not changed these requirements much (see Chapters 5 and 6 for more information).

While the JCAHO used to require a medical staff policy statement regarding restraint (typically located in the medical staff rules and regulations), its new standards mention a plan and imply the need for a series of policies, procedures, and protocols. Even organizations that complied with the pre-1996 JCAHO standards likely needed to do additional work to comply with the 1996 standards. Medical and surgical facilities that comply with the 1996 standards should review their policies, since JCAHO requirements for them have actually become somewhat less restrictive. A medical and surgical facility with a psychiatric unit must have either two different restraint policies or a single policy that provides for the two different sets of requirements.

The following sections discuss the history and current roles of various types of documents relating to restraint. Guidelines for a plan and a set of policies and procedures are also included to help organizations develop their own documents.

Bylaws

To comply with JCAHO requirements, all hospitals must have two sets of bylaws: the bylaws of the board or the governing body (as the JCAHO calls it) and the bylaws of the medical staff.

The governing body bylaws establish the ownership and governance of the hospital, and they usually do not deal at all with clinical matters. They usually include a provision for the medical staff to be a semiautonomous body that organizes and governs itself through its own bylaws.

The medical staff bylaws often contain some discussion of clinical matters. The JCAHO used to require medical staff bylaws or rules and regulations (see below) to deal with restraint, so some organizations' medical staff bylaws still do. But today, the JCAHO no longer requires medical staff bylaws to cover restraint, although it still considers this acceptable.

However, it is not a good idea for medical staff bylaws to deal with such detailed clinical matters as restraint because it can be quite difficult to reach an agreement quickly on details and make changes to the bylaws when clinical practices change. Bylaws changes usually require the approvals of the medical executive committee (MEC), the medical staff (at an official meeting convened after sufficient official notice), and the board, so it is not uncommon for a change to take a year or more from start to finish. In the meantime, either clinical practice is not in accord with professional consensus, or clinical practice in the organization has changed but is not in compliance with the bylaws. If the bylaws are properly written to permit it, then the rules and regulations or medical staff policies are the best places to deal with those detailed clinical issues with which the medical staff is concerned. These documents can be changed far more easily and quickly than bylaws.

Rules and regulations

An organization's rules and regulations are a set of detailed guidelines, usually required in an organization's bylaws, that focus heavily on clinical subjects. (There does not seem to be any difference between a *rule* and a *regulation*, but the combined term is almost always used, perhaps by habit.)

Unlike bylaws, rules and regulations are relatively easy to change in most hospitals—requiring only a vote by the MEC—therefore, it is not a problem to include many details regarding clinical matters, such as restraint, in the rules and regulations. But because rules and regulations are basically intended for governing and guiding medical staff members (as are medical staff bylaws), an organization should be sure to include guidelines regarding issues that extend beyond medical staff members—as restraint does—in other documents as well.

Plan

Most organizations have one or more comprehensive documents called *plans* that outline, in detail, what they currently do and what they hope to do. The 1999 JCAHO standards require organizations to cover restraint in their plans or policies and procedures (TX.7.1.1.1 and TX.7.5 intent in the hospital standards).

Exactly which documents deal with restraint depends upon how the organization organizes its documents. Considering the importance of restraint and seclusion, it is certainly useful to devote some part of the clinical plan to that area. An organization's plan should provide an overview of the organization's approach, goals, allocation of resources, and monitoring of effectiveness regarding restraint use. An organization might find it simplest to place its planning document for restraint within its plan for provision of care (required by standard LD.3 in the Leadership chapter of the *Comprehensive Accreditation Manual for Hospitals [CAMH])*. (See Figure 7.1, p. 183, for a sample plan.)

Policies and procedures

An organization's policies and procedures—which are often combined into one document or are at least filed together even when they are in separate documents—outline how the organization's goals and approaches, as presented in its plan, are to be put into practice. Procedure statements relating to restraint, for example, present step-by-step descriptions of the responsibilities of each of the various types of healthcare personnel who carry out restraint. Each procedure statement is usually matched with a corresponding policy statement that presents the objectives and limits of restraint.

Department heads or similar officials usually review and approve policies and procedures, under the authority of the organization's CEO or medical staff president. Therefore, policies and procedures can be changed easily and quickly, as clinical practice requires. In most hospitals, the details of restraint use are specified in the policies and procedures of the nursing department and are sometimes repeated in the medical staff rules and regulations or in medical staff departmental policies (see above).

Policy and procedure statements vary widely among organizations because each organization's policies and procedures must be tailored to the characteristics of its patient group, the training and capabilities of personnel, community practice, and the physical characteristics of the facility. For this reason, Figure 7.2 (p. 188) does not offer detailed suggestions, but rather headings and brief descriptions of some of the procedure statements that an organization might wish to develop.

Protocols

A clinical protocol—sometimes referred to as an *algorithm,* a *practice guideline,* a *decision tree,* or a *preferred practice pattern*—is a published or officially recognized guideline for carrying out some clinical procedure. In the context of the JCAHO standards regarding restraint, protocol has a very specific and limited meaning: It is a document that—when approved by the medical staff, nursing leadership, and any other appropriate groups, such as administration—authorizes certain nurses to apply restraint without a licensed independent practitioner's order.

To be acceptable to the JCAHO, a restraint protocol must

- be applicable only within a clearly defined setting and for a specifically described group of patients;
- describe the set of symptoms or events (criteria) that trigger its applicability;
- outline the level of patient monitoring required during its application; and
- state the criteria for discontinuing its application.

An organization might maintain its set of protocols in a separate document or include them in its policies and procedures. But regardless of where protocols are contained, the medical staff must approve them. (See Figure 7.3, p. 189, for sample policies pertaining to restraint protocols.)

Acceptable protocols do not focus on the use of restraint. Instead, each protocol must deal with care of patients with a particular diagnosis or clinical problem or undergoing a particular procedure (for example, patients on a ventilator). The protocol should contain a series of steps for managing the patient, one of which is use of restraint if less restrictive alternatives failed to be effective. Therefore, the title of a protocol should never include the term restraint.

Protocols are not acceptable in behavioral healthcare settings (although the standards in the behavioral healthcare manual, which are the standards promulgated for hospitals in the 1996 revision, do discuss the use of protocols). However, a behavior management program developed by a properly qualified professional can permit restraint or seclusion without a doctor's order (see discussion of contingent restraint in Chapter 2). The behavior management plan is analogous to a protocol. At the time this book goes to press, JCAHO is discussing clarification of the definition and characteristics of an acceptable behavior management plan.

The samples provided in this chapter

JCAHO surveyors are generally not concerned with document titles or where documents are located; they look to see that necessary documents exist and have been properly approved. And, regarding restraint, with the exception of mental health settings, the JCAHO provides organizations with little guidance on the details of the various documents beyond specifying what they must contain, so an organization has a great deal of leeway in determining what meets its own needs. (The JCAHO is still quite prescriptive with its documentation requirements for mental health settings, so such organizations should consult the JCAHO's *Comprehensive Accreditation Manual for Behavioral Health Care* for more information on general documentation.)

The samples in this chapter are intended to assist an organization in developing its own plan, policies, and procedures for restraint use that comply with the new JCAHO standards. These samples are not complete documents but rather represent an outline that each facility will need to expand to mesh with its own patient mix, physical setting, and staffing pattern.

The samples provide a means that we believe will assist an organization in meeting JCAHO requirements. In some areas, the samples go considerably beyond what the JCAHO standards require because compliance alone does not ensure safe, appropriate restraint use. For example, the plan suggests that licensed independent practitioners be permitted to order restraint only after having received special training to do so, although the JCAHO does not require this.

There is no guarantee that any particular document will be found to be in compliance with the JCAHO standards when subject to survey. Even today, a certain amount of survey evaluation is subjective, and success depends upon convincing surveyors that compliance exists. The JCAHO effort to be nonprescriptive and allow organizations to develop the best methods to suit their individual situations, however, is a major change (see Chapter 5 for more discussion on the new JCAHO survey process). If an organization's plan, policies, and procedures are not in agreement with a surveyor's own clinical judgment or preferences, the surveyor will most likely defer to an organization's own documents if they have been appropriately considered and approved.

Figure 7.1

Sample Plan

Definitions

In this organization's plan and its related policies and procedures, the following definitions apply:

- Restraint: Any method of applying involuntary restriction on a patient's bodily movement or access to his or her body areas. This definition of restraint excludes restrictions that are inherent and customary parts of medical, dental, surgical, or diagnostic procedures and the use of devices whose main purpose is to provide postural support or to avoid direct, accidental injuries.

- Seclusion: Involuntary, solitary confinement of a patient (or confinement with only a staff observer present) in a room from which the patient is physically prevented from exiting.

Purpose and use of restraint

Restraint is a high-risk, potentially harmful procedure that is intended to be used only when less restrictive methods have not succeeded or clearly are not likely to succeed in preventing injury to a patient or others. Any application of restraint must involve consideration of the degree and likelihood of the harm that may be *prevented* by the restraint compared to the degree and likelihood of the harm that may be *produced* by the restraint. Restraint is to be applied for no longer than it is clearly needed, and any doubts about the need for restraint should be resolved in favor of using an alternative to restraint.

Undesirable effects of restraint

Restraint has been demonstrated to produce serious negative physical, psychological, and social effects, including skin lesions, overheating and dehydration, temporary or permanent incontinence, feelings of demoralization and humiliation, and temporary or permanent disruption of adult identity. In evaluating the applicability of restraint to any clinical situation, the patient's susceptibility to

Figure 7.1 **Sample Plan (continued)**

these effects must be taken into account. And when a patient is restrained, periodic observation of the patient's condition should include consideration of whether any of these undesirable effects is developing.

Even the use of restraint-like procedures or devices that are excluded as restraint by this organization's definition may still lead to the undesirable effects listed above. For this reason, patients whose movement is restricted but whose care is excluded from the application of restraint policies or procedures must nevertheless be observed for the development of undesirable effects.

Alternatives to restraint

Before each application of restraint, consideration must be given to the possibility of using an alternative method that is less dangerous and less restrictive than restraint. Available alternatives include

- increasing the intensity of nursing care;
- using family or friends to observe and occupy the patient;
- removing and subsequently reinserting any lines or tubes that a patient may be inclined to remove; and
- using mechanical or electronic signaling devices.

Restraint reduction program

Reducing the frequency of restraint use in this hospital is a high priority. All nursing staff members will receive a review of the available means of avoiding restraint use as part of their initial orientation and annual inservice training. Statistics regarding the frequency of restraint use and correlations between frequency and other variables will be collected and assessed at least monthly. And the information obtained from statistical reviews will be used to determine what measures are likely to be effective in reducing restraint use.

Figure 7.1. Sample Plan (continued)

Staff training

Only staff who are trained in applying restraints, monitoring restrained patients, and releasing patients from restraint will be involved in restraint related activities. Training for these roles will be provided to all nursing staff members as part of their initial orientation and annual inservice training. At least 50% of each training session will be devoted to the practical application of principles and to the use of various restraint devices to minimize danger to patients and staff. Staff who attend such training sessions will be required to complete a brief pencil-and-paper test to demonstrate that they understand the principles presented.

Assurance of staff competence

Staff members may not participate in the application, monitoring, or removal of restraint until they demonstrate competence in related decisions and tasks. Staff will be required to periodically demonstrate competence through testing at the completion of orientation and inservice training. Individual staff members might also be asked to take additional training or undergo testing if observations by supervisors or the occurrence of work-related incidents with patients suggest a need to do so.

Protection of patients' rights, dignity, and well-being

Because restraint use presents a danger to a patient's rights, dignity, and well-being, specific efforts must be taken to protect these. Patient rights must be protected by obtaining the consent of a patient or guardian before implementing restraint procedures whenever possible. Restraint must be applied humanely and as briefly as possible, and staff must keep in mind the danger restraint presents to a patient's self-esteem, feelings of independence, and pride. Staff must also exercise special care to avoid the negative physical and psychological effects of restraint, and they must meet all of a patient's essential needs during a restraint episode, including food, liquids, access to the toilet, exercise, and protection of skin. To the extent feasible, a patient's treatment program should continue during restraint, and the patient's participation in treatment should be facilitated.

Figure 7.1 **Sample Plan (continued)**

Use of protocols

In accordance with JCAHO standard TX.7.5.3.2, nurses may apply restraint under specific treatment protocols. Only a registered nurse who has completed required training and has demonstrated competence, however, may decide when a protocol is applicable.

Protocols may be adapted from published literature or written by nursing staff, but must be approved by the medical staff, nursing administration, and the vice president for clinical care. Protocols must also specify

- a specific patient group and a setting for applicability (ventilator patients in the ICU, for example);
- at which time intervals a patient's condition must be reassessed;
- the requirements regarding observation and documentation of a restrained patient; and
- criteria for discontinuing restraint use.

Use of orders to initiate restraint use

Only physicians who have received appropriate training relating to restraint and have been granted the privilege to order restraint can initiate restraint orders. Orders must state a specific length of time for which the restraint may apply—up to and including 24 hours (orders may not exceed 24 hours). A physician must personally complete a direct patient assessment to initiate a restraint order or to renew an order after 24 hours. Orders or accompanying progress notes must:

- state the justification for restraint;
- describe the unsuccessful attempt to use alternatives;
- describe the patient assessment; and
- include the criteria for releasing the patient from restraint.

Figure 7.1 **Sample Plan (continued)**

Performance improvement

Improvement of restraint use is a constant priority for this hospital's performance improvement system. Continuous measurement and assessment of the frequency of restraint use is a required activity, and appropriate measures are taken to improve performance.

Medical record documentation

Every use of restraint is to be documented in the patient's record. At a minimum, documentation must include

- the alternatives tried before restraint use;
- the justification for restraint;
- the patient assessment that demonstrates the need for restraint as part of the patient's treatment;
- the applicability of a protocol or a time-limited order by a licensed independent practitioner;
- evidence that shows monitoring of the patient's condition during restraint; and
- demonstration of the need for continuing restraint beyond the initial order or of the satisfaction of criteria for release.

The records of patients who were restrained must receive 100% review as part of the hospital's medical record review procedure.

Figure 7.2 **Sample Procedure Statements**

As noted above, because procedure statements vary widely among organizations, this figure does not contain detailed suggestions, but lists some of the procedure statements that an organization might wish to develop.

Assessment of patients at risk for restraint: details the assessment process and how to document examinations.

Emergency assessment of patients in need of restraint: details the emergency assessment process and how to document examinations.

Use of a clinical protocol: explains who is authorized to use a protocol, how to follow a protocol, and how to document use of a protocol.

Carrying out alternatives to restraint: discusses which alternatives are available, steps for using the alternatives, and how to document the use of alternatives.

Application of restraint: describes techniques for safely applying restraint in the various settings in which restraint might be used, such as the emergency department and medical units, and how to document restraint use.

Orders for restraint: details who may issue orders, who may receive telephone/verbal orders, who may respond to orders, and who may extend orders.

Release from restraint: details who may release patients, the criteria for release, and the steps to take after a patient is released.

Cleaning, storing, and maintaining restraint materials and devices: discusses infection control procedures, storage places and methods, and how to repair restraint materials and devices.

Monitoring and care of restrained patients: describes monitoring responsibilities, documentation, and attention to patient needs.

Concurrent review of each episode of restraint by nursing management: requires that each use of restraint be reported immediately to the senior nurse manager on duty, who must visit the restrained patient and review the documentation in the patient's record at least once before the end of the work shift.

Figure 7.3 **Sample Policies**

Definitions

Note: See the restraint and seclusion plan in Figure 7.1 for definitions of restraint and seclusion.

- Patient needs: the physiological and psychological needs that a restrained or secluded patient requires to protect his or her well-being, dignity, and comfort. A nurse may determine a patient's needs based on the needs of average patients or on an assessment of the patient, whichever seems most effective in the situation. Physiological needs include at least liquids, food, toilet access, skin integrity, circulatory well-being, bathing, and limb movement. Psychological needs include human interaction, respect for dignity and well being, and information about the treatment situation.

- Protocol: an appropriately approved directive for the nursing staff that consists of a set of standardized criteria, clinical steps, and procedures for treating a condition or set of symptoms that can include applying restraint after the failure of less restrictive alternatives, and often a set of specifications for terminating the use of restraint.

- Voluntary use: the use of procedures such as restraint or seclusion with a patient who consents to their use. The patient must be legally capable of consenting (of appropriate mental capacity and age) and must receive sufficient information about the procedure to be able to weigh the pros and cons and arrive at an informed decision.

- Medical immobilization: the use of a device that is routinely or inherently part of a medical, surgical, dental, or diagnostic procedure that immobilizes a patient or restricts a patient's access to part of his or her body.

Figure 7.3 **Sample Policies (continued)**

- Adaptive support: the use of a device that compensates for muscular or skeletal weakness and assists a patient in assuming or maintaining normal posture.

- Medical protective device: a device that prevents accidental injury due to temporary loss of consciousness or diminished alertness usually resulting from a treatment procedure—not from permanent cognitive dysfunction or deliberate misbehavior.

- Behavior management: a systematic program in which a plan prepared by a competent psychological specialist is used to increase the frequency of desirable behavior and to reduce the frequency of undesirable behavior through specific positive and negative reinforcers.

- Adequate clinical justification: a listing and discussion of symptoms and other behaviors that indicate that despite possible negative consequences, restraint use is necessary.

- Assessed needs: the elements of a patient's current clinical condition—revealed through the patient's medical history and mental and physical evaluations—that substantiate restraint use.

- Forensic or correctional patients: patients who are in the custody of police or correctional authorities, as opposed to patients who are simply transported by police as a courtesy or are brought in for medical evaluation but are not in custody.

- Limited, justified use of restraint: the application of restraint only to the extent required when less restrictive methods and preventive attempts fail to be effective in dealing with behavior that clearly endangers the life or physical well-being of a patient or others.

- Qualified staff (those who are authorized to use restraint protocols): Registered nurses who complete the hospital-sponsored training program

Figure 7.3 **Sample Policies (continued)**

and pass the examination on use of restraint protocols. The names of all qualified staff members must appear on the official list of qualified staff.

- Competent, trained staff (those who are authorized to apply restraints and monitor and release restrained patients): patient care staff who complete the hospital-sponsored training program and pass both the written and practical examinations on how to apply restraint, release from restraint, and monitor restrained patients and whose personnel files contain evidence of such.

- Licensed, qualified, and authorized staff (those who are authorized to reassess restrained behavioral health patients and continue restraint orders): registered nurses who are employed as charge nurses or nurse managers for the psychiatric unit who complete the hospital-sponsored training program and pass the examination on reassessing restrained patients and evaluating the need for continuation of restraint.

Use of immobilizing or restraining devices for purposes other than restraint
Devices that are commonly used to restrain patients or restrict patients' freedom of movement or access to their own bodies may be used for medical immobilization, adaptive support, or accident prevention. Patients who are competent to consent to the use of such devices frequently do so. But even without consent, the JCAHO waives the applicability of its standards to the use of a device that meets the definition in this set of policies.

When the use of a device for some purpose other than restraint is not an inherent part of a medical procedure, its use must be documented in the patient's record, and the documentation must substantiate that the purpose of the device is not restraint. Even when a device is not used for restraint, however, regular periodic attention to the patient's needs must be carried out and documented on the appropriate form.

Figure 7.3 **Sample Policies (continued)**

Prevention of restraint/alternatives to restraint

The policy of this hospital is to reduce the frequency of restraint use to the greatest extent possible. To that end

- alternatives to restraint use will be developed as quickly as possible and will be continuously monitored for effectiveness and opportunities for further development;
- medical and nursing personnel will attempt to use one or more less-restrictive alternatives before each use of restraint; and
- if restraint use is necessary even after less restrictive alternatives are tried, personnel will document in the patient's record which alternatives were explored.

The alternatives that are usually appropriate for dealing with behaviors that might trigger restraint are

- patient education on the importance of the medical procedures, to encourage cooperation;
- regular removal and reinsertion of lines, tubes, and catheters to avoid a patient's pulling them out;
- frequent visits by staff, family, or friends and other distractions to avoid a patient's removing lines or tubes, wandering, or getting out of bed without help;
- attaching alarms to a patient or to a patient's bed to prevent him or her from wandering or getting out of bed without help; and

Figure 7.3

Sample Policies (continued)

- using medication to reduce anxiety, distractibility, antagonism, or hostility.

Use of restraint protocols by nursing personnel

Registered nurses who have completed the training and testing required to use restraint protocols are authorized to initiate restraint use in accordance with the criteria and procedures stated in the appropriate protocol. (Protocols are located in the nursing policy book.) When restraint is applied via protocol, nurses must be sure to meet all requirements regarding restraint—including patient and family education and protection of the patient's rights, dignity, and well-being—that are outlined elsewhere in relevant plans and policies.

After assessing a patient and determining that the patient requires restraint and meets the criteria stated in a protocol, a nurse must document the following

- the assessment;
- evidence that the patient meets the criteria in the protocol;
- the placement of the patient in restraints;
- the monitoring of the patient and attention to the patient's needs;
- periodic re-evaluations for the need to continue restraint; and
- the time at which the patient met the criteria for release from restraint, as outlined in the protocol.

Figure 7.3 **Sample Policies (continued)**

Each protocol may remain in effect for only a limited number of hours (as stated in each protocol). If a patient still needs restraint when a protocol expires, nurses must consult a physician to obtain an order for restraint, which may be an order to renew the protocol. When a patient whom a nurse restrains via protocol meets the protocol's criteria for release from restraint, the nurse must release the patient from restraint. If a patient appears to need reapplication of a restraint and meets protocol criteria after he or she is released from a restraint, the nurse may reapply restraint.

Physicians' orders for restraint

Any physician member of the active medical staff who is privileged to do so may issue an order for restraint. Before writing an order for restraint (or immediately after an emergency application of restraint), a physician must conduct a face-to-face assessment of the patient and do cument that the patient requires use of restraint and that no less restrictive alternative has been or is likely to be effective. Orders must be in writing and are good for up to 24 hours. Should a patient continue to need restraint beyond 24 hours, a physician must conduct a face-to-face evaluation before issuing a new order.

For emergency situations in which no physician is present, a registered nurse may direct that a patient must be placed in restraint, but must immediately contact the appropriate physician to request a telephone order. When a patient is restrained via protocol and still needs restraint at the expiration of the protocol, a physician must carry out a face-to-face evaluation before writing an order to continue restraint.

RESOURCE GUIDE

The following pages list and describe some of the most important and useful published articles and books relating to restraint and seclusion. Many of them focus on restraint in long-term care settings, but are nevertheless relevant for use in other settings. Although there are relatively few published objective, quantitative studies regarding restraint and seclusion use, we believe that we have found most of them. Readers who are interested in doing a more extensive review of available information on restraint and seclusion will find useful leads to literature in the bibliographies of several of the articles listed on the following pages. In addition, this resource guide includes the names and addresses of two organizations that offer literature and other materials relating to restraint and seclusion.

Articles

Barr, Wendy. 1996. Do Restraints Really Protect Intubated Patients? *Am. J. Nursing* 96(6):51. *A brief review of several recent articles that suggest that restraint of intubated patients may be useless or harmful, and describes measures that may be used instead of restraint.*

Betemps, Elizabeth, et al. 1993. Hospital Characteristics, Diagnoses, and Staff Reasons Associated with Use of Seclusion and Restraint. *Hosp. & Commun. Psychiat.* 44:367-371. *Statistical analysis of restraint and seclusion use in 82 VA hospitals.*

Capezuti, Elizabeth, et al. 1996. Physical Restraint Use and Falls in Nursing Home Residents. J. *Am. Ger. Soc.* 44:627-633. *A statistical study of nursing home residents that shows that residents who were restrained had a higher chance of falling than those who were not restrained. This report does not prove anything, but is suggestive.*

Crenshaw, Wesley and Francis, Paul. 1995. A National Survey on Seclusion and Restraint in State Psychiatric Hospitals. *Psychiatric Services* 46:1026-1031. *A survey of 101 state hospitals in 44 states that reveals considerable variation in use of restraint and seclusion, suggesting lack of agreed-upon standards for use.*

Evans, Lois and Strumpf, Neville. 1989. Tying Down the Elderly: A Review of the Literature on Physical Restraint. *J. Am. Ger. Soc.* 37:65-74. *A general overview of what is known about the pros and cons of restraint use.*

Fisher, William. 1994. Restraint and Seclusion: A Review of the Literature. *Am. J. Psychiat.* 151:1584-1591. *A review of the literature on restraint and seclusion use, from the perspective of psychiatric hospitals, that describes pros and cons and includes suggestions for improvement.*

Frengley, J.D. 1986. Influence of Physical Restraints on Acute General Medical Wards. *J. Am. Ger. Soc.* 34:565-568. *A study of patients admitted to acute, general medical wards that shows that 7.4% of all patients and 20.3% of those 70 years of age or older were restrained at some time.*

Kane, Robert, et al. 1993. Restraining Restraints: Changes in a Standard of Care. *Ann. Rev. Publ. Hlth.* 14:545-84. *An extensive review of changing attitudes regarding restraint use in long-term care facilities.*

Kapp, Marshall. 1992. Nursing Home Restraints and Legal Liability: Merging the Standards of Care and Industry Practice. *J. Legal Med.* 13:1-32. *A review of the legal issues relating to restraint in nursing homes, much of which is relevant to use in acute care as well.*

Lofgren, Richard, et al. 1989. Mechanical Restraints on the Medical Wards: Are Protective Devices Safe? *Am. J. Publ. Hlth.* 79:735-738. *A prospective study of restrained patients admitted to a general medical ward in a VA hospital that shows that 6% of admittees were restrained and that patients restrained for more than four days had relatively high rates of nosocomial infections and pressure sores.*

Marks, Wayland. 1992. Physical Restraints in the Practice of Medicine. Arch. Intern. Med. 152:2203-2206. *A brief review of restraint use in long-term and acute care, emphasizing the negative effects and the use of alternatives. The review notes that there is no evidence of the efficacy of restraints.*

Mion, Lorraine, et al. 1989. A Further Exploration of the Use of Physical Restraints in Hospitalized Patients. *J. Am. Ger. Soc.* 37:949-956. *A study of 421 patients admitted to a general medical ward or a rehabilitation medical ward that shows that 13% of the general medical patients were restrained and that 34% of the rehabilitation patients were restrained. Of the patients able to be interviewed, 33% expressed negative perceptions about restraint.*

Mion, Lorraine and Strumpf, Neville. 1994. Use of Physical Restraints in the Hospital Setting: Implications for the Nurse. *Geriatric Nursing* 15:127-132. *A review of key principles for nurses to reduce restraint use in general hospitals.*

Ray, Nancy and Rappaport, Mark. 1995. Use of Restraint and Seclusion in Psychiatric Settings in New York State. *Psychiatric Services* 46:1032-1037. *A survey of 125 psychiatric settings that shows great variations in frequency of restraint use among settings and that restraint use seems unrelated to the characteristics of the patient populations.*

Robbins, Laurence J. et al. 1987. Binding the Elderly: A Prospective Study of the Use of Mechanical Restraints in an Acute Care Hospital. *J. Am. Ger. Soc.* 35:290-296. *A direct observational study (i.e., not relying solely on chart reports) of medical and surgical patients admitted to a VA hospital that finds that 17% of patients were restrained at some point, but that of these patients, 38% had no record in their charts that restraint had been applied.*

Rubenstein, Howard, et al. 1983. Standards of Medical Care Based on Consensus Rather Than Evidence: The Case of Routine Bedrail Use for the Elderly. *Law, Medicine and Healthcare* 11:271-276. *This article discusses how bedrails may help or harm patients, but evidence is lacking despite common perceptions and practice.*

Rubin, Bruce, et al. 1993. Asphyxial Deaths Due to Physical Restraint: A Case Series. *Arch. Fam. Med.* 2:405-408. *Based on a mail survey of 37 death investigators who provided information on 63 deaths, this article shows that the majority of deaths occurred when restraints were correctly applied. Argues that restraints are inherently dangerous.*

Schnelle, John, et al. 1996. Editorial: To Use Physical Restraints or Not? *J. Am. Ger. Soc.* 44:727-728. *A critique of the study by Capezuti, et al. that points out that good objective research on the effects of restraints is needed.*

Books

Blumenreich, Patricia and Lewis, Susan (eds.). *Managing the Violent Patient: A Clinician's Guide.* Brunner/Mazel, 1993. *A collection of chapters dealing with many aspects of violent psychiatric patients. Since one of the major reasons for restraint and seclusion use in psychiatric facilities is to control violence, there is a good deal here that relates to restraint and seclusion.*

Braun, Judith and Lipson, Steven (eds.). *Toward a Restraint-Free Environment.* Health Professions Press, 1993. *A compilation of chapters that cover most of the major issues of restraint use. Although lacking some of the data and latest thinking that can be found in some journal articles, this is an excellent single document for an overview of the reasons and means to reduce restraint.*

Kendal Corporation. *Untie the Elderly: Resource Manual, Third Edition,* 1994. *Available from Kendal Corporation,* PO *Box* 100, *Kennett Square,* PA 19348. *A collection of key articles and training materials, presented mainly from a long-term care perspective, for organizations interested in reducing or eliminating restraint use.*

Robins, Natalie. The Girl Who Died Twice. Delacorte Press, 1995. *A narrative description of the treatment of a young woman in a major academic medical center that ended with the patient's death. It appears that inappropriate use of restraint had a major role in the unfortunate ending.*

Tardiff, Kenneth (ed.). *The Psychiatric Uses of Seclusion and Restraint.* American Psychiatric Press, 1984. *A collection of chapters by various authors on a variety of aspects of restraint and seclusion use. The emphasis is on theory rather than practical clinical discussion.*

Thackrey, Michael. *Therapeutics for Aggression: Psychological/Physical Crisis Intervention.* Human Sciences Press, 1987. *A discussion of the available means for dealing with dangerous patients in psychiatric settings, including details on how to use physical means to control patients.*

Organizations

Kendal Corporation, PO Box 100, Kennett Square, PA 19348. Phone: 610/388-5580. A not-for-profit organization that carries out the project "Untie the Elderly" in long term care facilities. It offers a variety of training materials, publications, and a free newsletter. Although the Kendal Corporation concentrates on long-term care, much of its material is useful for psychiatric and acute care facilities.

Posey Company, 5635 Peck Road, Arcadia, CA 91006. Phone: 800/44-POSEY. This company which is so well known and has been in the restraint business for so long that one of their devices is named after them offers a wide variety of restraint equipment, devices, and training materials.

Glossary

The following pages contain definitions for some of the key terms used in this book. Some of the terms come directly from the JCAHO standards or intent statements but are not defined by the JCAHO. Other terms are referred to or implied in the JCAHO standards.

These definitions have been prepared with several objectives in mind:

- to be easily incorporated into a hospital policy on restraint that complies with the JCAHO standards;
- to be used as part of a hospital policy that is practical and can be easily instituted; or
- to be used as part of a hospital policy or in staff training programs that are in accord with current professional practice.

State laws or regulations may include some definitions that overlap or contradict some of the following definitions, so as with every aspect of restraint or seclusion practice, readers should check local requirements before making any revisions. Some of these definitions may not be applicable in long-term care settings.

Adaptive support: the use of a device that compensates for muscular or skeletal weakness and assists a patient in assuming or maintaining normal posture.

Adequate clinical justification: a listing and discussion of symptoms and other behaviors that indicate that despite possible negative consequences, restraint use is necessary.

Assessed needs: the elements of a patient's current clinical condition—revealed through the patient's medical history and mental and physical evaluations—that substantiate restraint use.

Behavior management: a systematic program in which a plan prepared by a competent psychological specialist is used to increase the frequency of desirable behavior and reduce the frequency of undesirable behavior through specific positive and negative reinforcers.

Competent, trained staff (those who are authorized to apply restraints and monitor and release restrained patients): patient care staff who complete the hospital-sponsored training program and pass both the written and practical examinations on how to apply restraint, release from restraint, and monitor restrained patients and whose personnel files contain evidence of such.

Forensic or correctional: adjectives used to describe patients who are in the custody of police or correctional authorities, as opposed to patients who are simply transported by police as a courtesy or are brought in for medical evaluation but are not in custody.

Licensed, qualified, and authorized staff: staff members who are authorized by the state (registration for nurses is the functional equivalent of licensure), receive appropriate training, and are authorized either by individual name or position to carry out the function of extending restraint orders. (In behavioral healthcare settings, this category refers to those staff who are authorized to reassess restrained patients and extend restraint orders for up to 24 hours).

Licensed independent practitioner: a healthcare practitioner authorized by state law and by the individual hospital to practice independently *in the hospital* (i.e., without medical supervision). This category typically includes physicians, dentists, and podiatrists. In some states, members of other professions are permitted to practice independently in the hospital; and in most states, a number of professions are permitted to practice independently outside the hospital, providing ambulatory care.

Limited, justified use of restraint: the application of restraint only to the extent required when less restrictive methods and preventive attempts fail to be effective in dealing with behavior that clearly endangers the life or physical well-being of a patient or others.

Medical immobilization: the use of a device that is routinely or inherently part of a medical, surgical, dental, or diagnostic procedure that immobilizes a patient or restricts a patient's access to part of his or her body.

Medical protective device: a device that prevents accidental injury due to temporary loss of consciousness or diminished alertness usually resulting from a treatment procedure—not from permanent cognitive dysfunction or deliberate misbehavior.

Patient needs: the physiological and psychological needs that a restrained or secluded patient requires to protect his or her well-being, dignity, and comfort. A nurse may determine a patient's needs based on the needs of average patients or on an assessment of the patient, whichever seems most effective in the situation. These needs include at least liquids, food, toilet access, skin integrity, circulatory well-being, bathing, and limb movement.

Protocol: a directive for the nursing staff that consists of a set of standardized criteria, clinical steps, and procedures for applying restraint, and often a set of specifications for terminating the use of restraint. The medical staff and administration must approve all protocols.

Qualified staff (those who are authorized to use restraint protocols): registered nurses who complete the hospital-sponsored training program and pass the examination on use of restraint protocols. The names of all qualified staff members must appear on the official list of qualified staff.

Restraint: any method of applying involuntary restriction on a patient's bodily movement or access to his or her body areas. This definition of restraint excludes restrictions that are inherent and customary parts of medical, dental, surgical, or diagnostic procedures and the use of devices whose main purpose is to provide postural support or to avoid direct, accidental injuries.

Seclusion: involuntary, solitary confinement of a patient (or confinement with only a staff observer present) in a room from which the patient is physically prevented from exiting.

Voluntary use: the use of procedures, such as restraint or seclusion, with a patient who consents to their use. The patient must be legally capable of consenting (of appropriate mental capacity and age) and must receive sufficient information about the procedure to be able to weigh the pros and cons and arrive at an informed decision.